Theory of Coping Systems

Change in Supportive Health Organizations

Theory of Coping Systems

Change in Supportive Health Organizations

FRANCIS D. POWELL

Schenkman Publishing Company, Inc.
Cambridge, Massachusetts

Schenkman Publishing Company, Inc.
Cambridge, Massachusetts 02138

Library of Congress Catalog Card Number 75-24554

ACKNOWLEDGEMENTS

Many colleagues and associates in the United States and abroad have contributed ideas and personal support to the completion of this work. Only a few can be mentioned here. Among those who provided intellectual basis for the work during years of research at Harvard University were Talcott Parsons, Theodore Mills, Samuel Stouffer, Philip Slater, along with John Kosa, who facilitated the initiation of the present study. Financial support was supplied by a grant from the United States Public Health Service.

During early phases of the research at Boston College the personal contributions of Buford Rhea, Ritchie Lowry, Severyn Bruyn, Benedict Alper and Everett Hughes were substantial. Members of the faculty of the Boston College School of Nursing, headed by Dean Rita Kelleher, participated actively in the development of basic concepts underlying the research and in the articulation of research procedures. During that period valuable insights were also derived from the nursing comments of Esther Lucille Brown, Virginia Olesen and Alice Stueks, and from the sociological comments of Morris Schwartz and Irving Zola. The generous cooperation of the families and the staff in the clinics was essential, but all names used in the book have been altered to safeguard the anonymity of the individuals studied.

The data analysis and write-up, which were conducted at the Tavistock Institute of Human Relations, were greatly forwarded by the sensitive and constructive suggestions of Robert Rapoport, Colin Parkes, Eric Miller, Joseph Lella, and Anselm Strauss, and by the able assistance of Robert Ballagh and Margaret Napier.

Among research assistants from various universities who have contributed vitally to the progress of the work are John Capobianco, Stephanie Catalan, Loretta Gill, Norma Goldberger and Leo Gravel; Andrew Chester, Jeffrey Howard, Robert Karasek, Mary Ellen Lane, John O'Neill and Luke Reyschler. The capable assistance in computer analysis of Mary Hyde and Richard LaBrie, Donald Ferree and Eliot Smith at the Computing Center and the Center for the Behavioral Sciences of Harvard University is gratefully acknowledged.

Personal appreciation is due to Lillian Rubin, Anne Freedman and Earl Ostroff who wrestled with the wording on both sides of the Atlantic, and to Joseph Hozid and Sherwin Feinhandler for perceptive colleague comment during the final preparation of the manuscript.

To my wife who typed, struggled with the prose, and somehow "coped" and to our sons and daughters who endured parental distraction patiently, gratitude is affectionately expressed.

TABLE OF CONTENTS

LIST OF FIGURES

GRAPHS

(In the first year each clinic is systematically compared with the orthopedic clinic. Comparisons are then made between the first and second years for each clinic.)

CHAPTER I

CHANGE WITHIN COPING SYSTEMS

I-1. Supportive Coping Systems[1]

Coping systems are social networks which deal with stress-producing long-term problems; they deal with these problems by means of available resources. Supportive coping systems are social networks in which primary responsibility for dealing with problems is assumed by the problem bearers themselves. Resocializing coping systems assign primary responsibility for dealing with long-term problems to assisting specialists.[2]

[1] This discussion of types of coping systems parallels somewhat the approach of Glaser and Strauss. Cf. Barney G. Glaser and Anselm L. Strauss, *The Discovery of Grounded Theory: Strategies for Qualitative Research,* Chicago: Aldine Publishing Company, 1967.

[2] Coping systems take on the characteristics of the institutions serving them. Thus families and communities coping with long-term stress with the help of supportive institutions are designated as supportive coping systems. Families and communities coping with long-term stress with the help of resocializing institutions are designated as resocializing coping systems.

Aspects of the present discussion are based on Wheeler's analysis of formal socialization organizations. Cf. Stanton Wheeler, "The Structure of Formally Organized Socialization Settings," in O. Brim and S. Wheeler, *Socialization After Childhood: Two Essays,* New York: John Wiley, 1966.

Supportive coping systems are, for example, family and staff networks of probation departments, open prisons, halfway houses, therapeutic communities, drug institutes, community mental health centers and after-care programs which cope with long-term stress through social support.[3]

Resocializing coping systems include maximum security prisons, custodial mental institutions, tuberculosis hospitals, detention camps, reform schools and military academies. Insofar as such programs minimize the use of the resources of those immediately confronting the problems, they are deficient as coping systems.

An important type of supportive coping system is concerned with the care of children. Families are confronted with problems of their mentally retarded or physically handicapped children. Minority group children who are targets of broad societal prejudice or disprivilege are faced with a range of difficulties. Certain flexible educational institutions and neighborhood youth centers provide support to the primary resources of families and communities in coping with these difficulties.[4]

A unique variety of coping system involves families dealing with the stress of chronic children's illness. Such families avail themselves of the services of ambulatory pediatric departments while assuming primary responsibility themselves for the child's care. The characteristics of various chronic pediatric diseases pose specific issues of stress for these families in their coping processes, and it is some of these specific issues that we shall deal with in this book.

Children with diabetes must from an early age assume autonomy in understanding and managing the condition. The principal responsibility for this autonomy training rests with the family. The unusual demands placed upon the child and the family is a cause of long term stress. The pediatric staff, in its secondary capacity, attempts to provide appropriate support to families coping with these problems.

In chronic pediatric arthritis, the uncertain and degenerative nature of the illness requires dependency and trust in medical judgment. Family responsibility for primary ambulatory care thus revolves around the issues of dependency on the hospital in making treatment changes and of family acceptance of the long-term incurable illness.

[3] For a closely related analysis of institutional concern with long-range issues cf. M. Lefton and W. R. Rosengren, "Organizations and Clients: Lateral and Longitudinal Dimensions," *American Sociological Review,* XXXI (December, 1966), pp. 802-810.

[4] Network coordination between supportive institutions within the community is documented in the present research. Cf. below V-5 through V-9.

This acceptance and trust is supported through a responsive and emotionally channelled staff-family relationship.[5]

With the hereditary fatal illness of cystic fibrosis long-term grief, guilt and ambivalence are major stress producing forces. Ritualized exchanges between staff and families reinforce the family process of coping with these forces and with the intermittent despair that accompanies them.

I-2. Dynamic Factors in a Supportive Organization

The physical setting for staff-family contact within a supportive institution serves to reinforce the character of family management of various illnesses. Thus, in the context of ambulatory outpatient services, waiting room contacts between staff and families are used to foster family autonomy in the home related aspects of the illness. On the other hand the intimacy of the examination room is often used as a setting to support families' need for dependency and acceptance of illness.

Coping systems are characterized by the looseness of their boundaries. Not only do "boundary spanning" personnel[6] such as nurses reach into communities to provide support, but family networks penetrate the helping institutions to negotiate for satisfaction of their needs. Owing to uncertain technology, diffuse need and capricious political status, staff and families mingle as definers and providers of the help that is required to deal with long term stress.[7] Through this

[5] These tendencies accord with Mills' observations on the group process of "rechannelling energies and feelings associated with interpersonal relations into the collective spirit." Cf. T. M. Mills, *The Sociology of Small Groups,* Englewood Cliffs, N. J.: Prentice-Hall, 1967, pp. 83 ff.

[6] James D. Thompson, *Organizations in Action,* New York: McGraw-Hill, 1967.

[7] The coping systems approach adopts a cultural point of view somewhat parallel to that of functional theory. However, contemporary institutions assume a mechanistic and individualistic design in terms of contractual, short-run relationships. The fact that human experience is not lived discretely and individualistically but continuously and socially, brings families into conflict with mechanistically constructed institutions. Since supportive institutions (e. g., chronic ambulatory care units) depart from the mechanistic mode, they incur internal strains within the major organizational structure. Families exploit these strains, especially in liaison with the middle range staff of coping institutions (i. e. nurses, social workers, etc.). Cf. parallel work of P. Blau (*Dynamics of Bureaucracy,* Chicago: University of Chicago Press, 1955) and A. Etzioni (ed., *The Semi-Professions and Their Organizations: Teachers, Nurses, Social Workers,* New York: New York Free Press, 1969); cf. also Lefton

sensitive, focused process the resources of family and community networks are brought to bear on these long term problems.[8]

The emotional interplay between family members and helping personnel is an important aspect of social support. Among the patterns isolated in this interplay, affective channelling and affective restraint figure prominently.[9]

The empirical focus of the present research is the interaction of families and staff in a health organization serving as an agency of support for families with chronic pediatric health problems. A number of children's ambulatory health services provided a context for the study of families and staff and their related community network resources.[10]

I-3. Setting for the Study of Change

This analysis is based on research conducted at a large metropolitan pediatric hospital.[11] The data was drawn primarily from transcriptions of tape recordings of interactions between clinic nurses and families in four pediatric outpatient services: arthritis, diabetes, orthopedics and cystic fibrosis. The recordings were made by nurse observers during two periods of two weeks each. While recording verbal exchanges the observers noted the presence of hospital personnel, patients and family members, and checked the location and time of each interaction. Recorded interviews and informal conferences were held with clinic nurses and physicians and supervisory staff, who were asked to describe their roles and the problems that tended to arise in the clinics. These meetings along with the direct observations of research staff members were useful in interpreting the recorded data.[12]

During the period of study the outpatient department moved from an old small building, to new and expanded facilities with additional

and Rosengren, *op. cit.* Cf. T. Parsons, *The Social System,* New York: Free Press, 1951.

[8] Coping systems, insofar as they involve active exchange process between staff and clients in shaping institutions toward long-range goals have something in common with the "adaptive process system model" proposed by Buckley. Cf. W. Buckley, *Sociology and Modern Systems Theory,* Englewood Cliffs: Prentice-Hall, 1967, pp. 40 ff.

[9] Cf. discussion of affectivity in Appendix A, p. 199.

[10] Cf. Elizabeth Bott, *Family and Social Networks; Roles, Norms, and External Relationships in Ordinary Urban Families,* London: Tavistock Publications, 1964.

[11] This research was supported by a grant from the United States Public Health Service (PHS NU00147).

[12] These clinic interviews were supplemented by a limited sample of structured interviews with families in their homes. These home contacts were use-

medical areas and large comfortable waiting rooms. With the move, additional clerical and nursing personnel were introduced to assist staff members in administrative and technical duties. In some instances the staff of physicians was also augmented. The first wave of observations was made just prior to the move from the old facilities, and the second took place seven months after the move. These observations have been supplemented by interviews and informal contacts with the clinics over a period of years. Follow-up contacts tend to substantiate the continuity of change in health service observed in connection with this organizational restructuring.

I-4. Nursing Focus and Coping Systems

Although the data from the outpatient departments included interactions with physicians and other members of the staff of the outpatient departments, the principal focus was the interaction between nurses and families. The broad range of roles involved provided a basis for the analysis of the outpatient services as coping institutions.

The centrality of nursing behavior in the data was useful as a means of gauging change in the outpatient clinics viewed as supportive institutions within coping systems. This research and parallel studies suggest that clinic nurses, social workers and community trained personnel are best equipped to support family coping processes; they are more identified with the personalized needs of families or communities,[13] than are neutral value-oriented, specialized autonomous professionals.[14] Physicians, institutionally backed bureaucrats and academi-

ful in assessing the quality of clinic health services delivered to families. Cf. Home Interview Questionnaire in Appendix C. Cf. Appendix A on methodology where procedures are described by which the recordings were reduced through numerical coding for computer analysis. Procedures by which the interactive process was analyzed sequentially are also described in that section of the report.

[13] Cf. Etzioni, *The Semi-Professions and Their Organizations,* on the variations from professional value orientation of nurses, teachers and social workers and the relevance of these variations for the human problems with which they are involved. Cf. also Etzioni *et al.* for a critical analysis of the Weberian type professional values as related to treatment of complex human problems.

[14] Cf. E. Freidson for a discussion of "non-autonomous consultants" and their relation to the "professions", in *Professional Dominance: The Social Structure of Medical Care,* New York: Atherton Press, 1970. Cf. also E. C. Hughes, *Men and Their Work,* New York: Free Press of Glencoe, 1958, for discussion of autonomy in the professionalizing process. See also Freidson and Hughes on the special case of the academic profession in regard to the issue of autonomy. In the present research the absence of professional autonomy on

cally trained behavioral science practioners, often have a professional incapacity for dealing with long range stress problems. The psychoanalytic "hour" is one classic example of a rational approach to the non-rational needs characteristic of long range situations. But nurses and social workers, though inspiring a lower level of expectation through a more muted image, are more generally in tune with the problems confronted by coping systems.[15]

the part of nurses was an important factor in family ability to mobilize hospital service on its behalf.

[15] Such inspiration of response in systems coping with long-term stress requires appropriate levels of reserved and expressed feelings made available to the ego during exchanges between families and staff. The intra-psychic forces required for such supportive interactive sequences are explained by Hartman and Kris.

Heinz Hartman ("Notes on the Theory of Sublimation", *Psycho-Analytic Study of the Child,* Vol. X, New York: 1954) expands Freud's definition of sublimation to include neutralization: the change of both libidinal and aggressive energy away from the instinctual and toward a noninstinctual mode. He thus equates neutralization with deinstinctualization and calls it the most important single factor in sublimation which makes achievement and the avoidance of repression possible.

The discharge of neutralized energy is the result of artistic inspiration (Ernst Kris, *Psychoanalytic Explorations in Art,* New York: Schocken Books, 1964) in which the ego relaxes to permit interplay with the id. This is a controlled regression, however, in which the degree of completeness of neutralization indicates the degree of ego autonomy. The perception of art differs from its creation in that the psychic shifts experienced by the viewer proceed from the consciousness, but the ego regression of the artist stems from preconscious thoughts which his ego permits to reach consciousness in an aesthetic disguise. In inspiration, the ego regresses but retains autonomy and through neutralized energy can achieve a desired creative result, whereas in fantasy, the ego processes are largely in the service of the id which intrudes upon the ego functions and inhibits aesthetic expression.

The psychoanalytic model to the extent that it assumed the dominance of the "id", is deterministic and "rational". To the extent to which the "ego" is seen as independent of the "id" and an "original source" through which new problems and interests can enter the psyche, the course of the life cycle becomes indeterminate and "non-rational". The Erikson model examines the life cycle in terms of "issues" and accepts indeterminacy and the predictively "non-rational". Erikson, in introducing cultural slanting to life cycle issues, rejects radical determinism.

Cf. S. Freud, "The Instincts and Their Vicissitudes" and "Group Psychology and the Analysis of the Ego," *The Standard Edition of the Complete Psychological Works of S. Freud,* London: Hogarth Press, 1971. Cf. also E. H. Erikson, *Identity and the Life Cycle in Psychological Issues,* Vol. 1, No. 1, New York: International Universities Press, 1959.

The aptness of particularistic, non-autonomous professionals such as nurses and social workers for supportive roles within coping systems, suggests a social variance rather than a social deviance model for such systems.[16]

The families involved in the present research appear to have coped more by varying in relation to accepted social norms than by deviating from these norms. Families with chronically ill children vary by assuming different life styles through hyper-individuation, rather than by directly challenging relevant social rules.[17]

I-5. A Typology for Analysis of Change

The analysis is based typologically on support settings which are either unicentered or polycentered. Unicentric settings highlight staff-based areas, while polycentric settings encompass both staff and family areas, and are designated as family-based. The typology is also differentiated in terms of ritual and improvisational interactive patterns.

From these locational and interactive components we derive four types of supportive coping organizations: staff-based improvisational, family-based improvisational, staff-based ritual and family-based ritual organizations.[18] Each corresponds empirically to one of the four outpatient clinics explored.[19]

[16] This social variance approach is parallel to the analysis of deviance as part of the "variety pool". The response of staff in giving support to the varied family coping styles suggests that the clinics tended to amplify and reinforce the coping methods evolved by families in coping with problems. Cf. Walter Buckley, *Sociology and Modern Systems Theory,* Englewood Cliffs, N. J.: Prentice Hall, 1967, pp. 166 ff. The social variation manifested by families and communities in coping systems suggests the "heterogeneous" environments discussed by Thompson. Contact with such "heterogeneous" contexts, according to Thompson, calls for the assignment of prominent functions to "boundary-spanning" and "discretionary" personnel and for a closely monitored social environment. In the present research such "boundary spanning" and discretionary monitoring of varied social environments was carried on by nursing personnel. Cf. Thompson, *Organizations in Action.*

[17] Cf. M. Voysey, "Official Agents and the Legitimation of Suffering," *Sociological Review,* NS XX (November, 1972), pp. 533-551. Cf. also discussion of social deviance and social control by T. Parsons in *Family, Socialization and Interaction Process Analysis,* New York: Free Press of Glencoe, 1955. Also, Parsons, *The Social System.*

[18] This typology resembles that developed by Perrow for task structures. The present analysis, however, views cultural, political and interactive factors as more independent of technology than does that of Perrow. Cf. Charles Perrow, "A Framework for the Comparative Analysis of Organizations," *American Sociological Review,* XXXII (April, 1967), pp. 194-208.

[19] The typology combines elements of ecological analysis as proposed by

The establishment of a basis for the interpretation of change within coping systems is a main interest in this typology. Health services characterized by improvisational interaction adapt more readily to increased bureaucratic complexity and to change in the institutional setting; those with ritual patterns are disrupted by such alterations. Institutional discrepancies foster the emergence of improvisational patterns of interaction. Improvising support systems in turn make use of such discrepancies to adapt positively to change. (See Figure A-I-5 for a schematic analysis of change in supportive coping systems.)

FIGURE A-1-5

SCHEMA FOR THE ANALYSIS OF CHANGE WITHIN COPING SYSTEMS

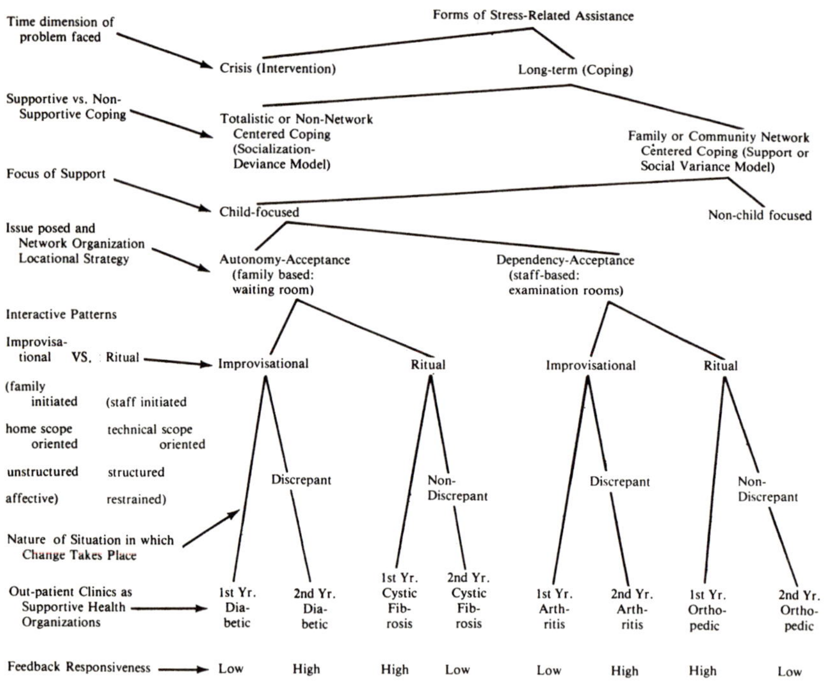

Rosengren and De Vault with an interactive approach to institutions dealing with long-term stress. Cf. W. R. Rosengren and S. De Vault, "The Sociology of Time and Space in an Obstetrical Hospital," in Eliot Freidson, ed., *The Hospital in Modern Society*, New York: The Free Press, 1963, pp. 266-291.

CHAPTER II

THE ARTHRITIS CLINIC: A STAFF BASED IMPROVISING ORGANIZATION

II-1. General Description of the Clinic

The arthritis services were provided within the facilities of the orthopedic department of the hospital. By virtue of this arrangement the arthritic clinic, though small in size, enjoyed the power and prestige associated with the surgical departments.

Despite its privileged position, there were substantial problems. A shortage of medical staff was compounded by the absence of the chief of the orthopedic services, which depressed morale and created confusion in the clinic's operation.

Although a special time was set aside one day a week for families with arthritic children, some families were obliged to receive treatment during general orthopedic clinic hours. The clinic was criticized by the head nurse who described its services as "poorly organized." However, parents expressed favorable views about the arthritic service of the hospital, despite these organizational problems. Lack of organization was compensated for by informal contact between families and staff. Families expressed their appreciation of the staff and spoke of friendships with other families making use of the clinic. While this view was not shared by the nursing staff, the informal atmosphere helped families make contact with each other and with staff members.

II-2. Physical and Organizational Structure of the Arthritis Services

Despite these opportunities for casual meeting there were considerable inconveniences. The arthritis services used the same facilities allocated to the general orthopedic department in a century-old outpatient building.[1] These consisted of a small grey waiting room about thirty feet by twenty-five in size, with wooden benches lining the walls along with a few tables displaying literature relating to the care of orthopedic and arthritic conditions. Adjoining the waiting room were three examination rooms and a forty foot corridor, at the entrance to which stood the administration desk of the clinic clerk. Further down the corridor were a physicians' office, a cast room, a laboratory, and a wash room for patients. (See Figure B-III-1, p. 34.)

For those children whose appointments fell within the special time allotted to arthritis families, these facilities were physically adequate. These families, however, often encountered shortages of physicians whose services were required elsewhere. Because of the absence of aides and the shortage of administrative help nurses were frequently interrupted during family interviews to run errands for physicians. There was little opportunity for nurses to consult with clinic notes or with other members of the staff and thus plan interviews. Contacts with arthritis families were almost totally unstructured. Absence of planning resulted in dependency on physicians and the staff nurse often functioned as a mere assistant to doctors in the examination rooms.

The nurse's role as doctors' assistant was especially prominent in cases where arthritis services were provided in conjunction with the general orthopedic clinic. Due to crowded conditions, interviews with these families were routine and rather brief.

The poor state of the clinic's service was reflected in the fact that only 57.5% of nursing time was spent with families during the first period of the research. This exceeded only the time spent in orthopedics, and was less than that devoted to family contact in diabetes and cystic fibrosis.[2]

II-3. Nature of the Illness and Treatment Approach

The patterns of behavior in the arthritis clinic were related to the nature of the illness itself and to the organization of treatment. Arthritis was notable for its chronic character. The chronicity of the condition was aggravated by its degenerative trend, its complexity and its unpre-

[1] The formal periods of observation occurred several years prior to the present report, and data gathered at that time has been supplemented by interviews with clinic staff.

[2] Cf. Appendix B, Table X, indicating that nursing time spent with families was 64.6% in diabetic, 62.0% in cystic fibrosis, and 43.6% in orthopedic.

dictability. The illness frequently involved related problems, as in rheumatoid arthritis, these complications occasioning deeper anxiety to family members and staff in dealing with the difficulties of the children.

Behavior in the clinic was also related to the manner in which medical treatment was carried out. Although routine treatment, such as the management of exercise and administration of drugs, was expected of the family, the regulation of care was closely controlled by the staff physicians. Any change in procedure required explicit medical direction. Changes in the condition that called for hospital decisions proved a source of worry to families. Parents often expressed their irritation at difficulties in contacting the medical staff when problems arose.

The incomplete medical control over arthritis gave rise to many problems in managing the disease. The changing symptoms and alterations of treatment procedures led to great uncertainties, referred to as the "put-off" nature of the illness. Parents and children were constantly "put-off" as to what to expect in treatment and in the social patterning of their lives.

Although the course of the illness was uncertain, the symptoms in most cases were ameliorable by appropriate medical procedures. It was impossible to anticipate precisely the problems that would arise, but an expectation existed that the staff would provide a remedy. Thus a wide range of problems marked family interviews. In addition to physical troubles, social and psychological issues touching on the illness were broached by families. Thorough acquaintance with the clinic and its ways facilitated the raising of home problems by families, many of whom had been visiting the hospital over a period of years.

II-4. Family Initiative

The nature of the illness and the limitations in medical control, caused a distinctive pattern of interaction to emerge. There was a tendency for discussion of problems to be initiated by families, rather than by the staff.[3] This tendency was due to sudden changes in the symptoms, shifts in treatment procedures, and the wide range of other problems involved, all factors related to the uncertainties of the condition.

Illness and treatment irregularities were magnified by organizational difficulties. Absence of planning of family interviews meant that the course of discussion was largely determined by the families themselves.

[3] Thus families showed higher rates of initiation than was recorded in any of the other clinics. Cf. Appendix B, Table II, showing 44.3% family initiation as compared with 36.7% in orthopedic, 36.4% in cystic fibrosis and 28.5% in diabetic.

Moreover, a rapid turnover in the medical staff resulted in the need for families to orient physicians and nurses as to the condition of the child, who quite often had been seen on previous visits by different staff members.

II-5. Family Anxiety and Staff Response

There was a tendency for the problems raised by families to have a social-emotional emphasis. The chronicity of the condition and the degenerative trend were powerful factors influencing family anxiety. The limited effectiveness of treatment procedures was a cause of worry. Uncertainty as to what procedures would be followed for increases in pain or stiffness in the joints also was a constant source of concern.

These difficulties were related to various anxiety patterns displayed by the staff in attempting to assist families. The anxiety of the nurse was reflected in frequent references to the authority of medical science and to the physicians of the hospital, references aimed at assuring families of medical control over the illness.[4] These assurances partly served to quiet nurses' fears about the child's condition. The anxiety of families was compounded by the need to make sudden independent decisions in the face of crises connected with the illness. The fact that such decisions were sometimes incorrect from a medical point of view gave rise to feelings of guilt, feelings which were especially difficult for the staff to handle.

The pattern of behavior displayed by the staff in response to family anxieties was somewhat ambivalent. There was an initial tendency to avoid responding to family social and emotional issues; nurses were ill-prepared to face these problems. Families, however, were able to apply pressure which made it very difficult not to respond.

The ability of some families to overcome staff reluctance was due to their familiarity with some of the personnel as a result of long periods of contact with the clinic. Personal acquaintance with physicians and nurses placed a claim upon the staff that called for some form of reassurance. Thus initial reluctance yielded to an effort by the staff to show understanding and encouragement for families in their struggles with the child's condition.

II-6. Social Networks and the Arthritis Association

The attendance, at regular clinic sessions, of a small number of families, many of whom had come to know each other, contributed to a

[4] Cf. figures on high arthritis rates of pronoun references to physicians, Appendix B, Table XIV, Col. 4. Over the two periods of observation, mothers referred to physicians by use of third person pronouns approximately once in every eighteen lines (17.96). This frequency was exceeded only by families with

sense of solidarity, which increased their ability to make claims upon the hospital. This solidarity was reinforced by membership in local chapters of the arthritis association. Families who were active in the association were able to make their demands known to the staff and to gain appropriate attention to their needs. Association families were able to define their roles as partial insiders in the hospital. They were able to reduce their sense of isolation within the medical system and influence the staff in achieving desired responses.

Membership in the community arthritis association provided an independent constituency for families, separate from the power structure of the hospital itself. The association also provided rapport among families and staff during visits to the hospital. This combination of inside and outside network leverage was effective in obtaining from the staff a response to family needs.[5]

II-7. Staff Based Family Contact

The staff-based character of the clinic was seen in that the principal point where contact with families took place was the examination room. The use of this area reflected the preference expressed by the arthritis nurse. In response to inquiries by a nursing assistant who was being oriented to clinic duties, the staff nurse expressed strong misgivings about the value of the waiting room as a location for family contact. According to the nurse, they preferred to "have that door shut" when discussing the personal problems of their children. In a similar vein the nurse expressed disapproval of group teaching during clinic visits for families having comparable problems. The practice of meeting each family separately in the privacy of the examination room represented a staff ideal of individualized treatment, and was regarded as expressing the wishes of the families themselves.

To a certain degree the data gathered on examination room interaction between staff and families validated these assumptions. In a number of cases families made forceful use of the examination room situation to present difficulties encountered in their attempts to deal with the illness of their children. Some families assumed a dominant position during examination room sequences. There were instances where

scolesosis problems (with a rate of one such physician reference every 10.39 lines).

[5] Membership in the arthritis association provided "organizational permeability to outside interests" suggested by Craig and Gross as a condition for "forum democracy". Cf. John Craig and Edward Gross, "The Forum Theory of Organizational Democracy: Structural Guarantees of Time-Related Variables," *American Sociological Review*, XXXV (February, 1970), pp. 19-33. Cf also E. Bott, *Family and Social Networks.*

families seized the initiative from the very beginning of the interaction and maintained control of the content and treatment of topics throughout.

The fact that the nurse usually was not able to formulate the agenda prior to family conferences reinforced family dominance. Due to this uncertainty, the examination room provided a distinct advantage to families in maintaining the initiative. The general lack of organization within the clinic and the exclusive attention that families could demand in the examination room made it relatively difficult for the staff to evade or avoid problems.[6]

II-8. An Example of Association Family Initiative

An example of family initiative in the examination rooms of the arthritis clinic was presented by a father and mother and their ten-year-old daughter. The child was suffering from a crippling condition and had to attend the clinic on crutches. The family was active in the arthritis association in their local community and participation in this organization figured prominently in the discussion that took place with the nurse. After an initial introduction, during which the nurse and mother discussed the efforts of the child to lose weight by closer adherence to her diet, the father interrupted by pointing out an article about the family that had been published in the journal of the local arthritis association.

Father to nurse: Look at this. This is the Arthritic Association of our home state. They made, they put a circular out, see.

Nurse to child: You were pretty fat, weren't you? [Mother laughs.]

Child to nurse: Yes.

Mother to nurse: You should have seen her around Christmastime. I think her waistline was bigger than mine. Not that I'm fat. [Child laughs nervously.]

Nurse to mother: But for ten years old . . . I think you're being practical about it. [Mother makes an inaudible comment, apparently referring to the child's weight.]

Father to nurse (showing more pictures): Here's another one. This was in the Arthritic Association paper.

Nurse to father: Aha.

[6] This family control parallels Rosengren and De Vault's analysis of patient delivery room behavior. Cf. Rosengren and De Vault, "The Sociology of Time and Space in an Obstetrical Hospital," in Freidson, ed., *The Hospital in Modern Society*, p. 285.

Father to nurse: And that's Julia in bed, see, with her cast on.

Mother to father and nurse: Yes. And this is the write-up in our paper.

Nurse to mother: Yes.

Mother to nurse: See how wonderful it was . . . in column 1?

Nurse to mother: Yes.

Mother to nurse: That's the Westport Times, that's what we . . .

Nurse (interrupting mother): Aha.

Mother to nurse: That's Westport.

Father to nurse: On account of they put that in, they write it up in the paper.

Mother to nurse: They called me up right away for the . . . the guy wanted to come up about 8 or 9:30. I don't know—8 or 9. I told him that was too early for me, brother, he stayed about two hours.

Father to nurse: That's quite a write-up, there, isn't it, there?

Mother to nurse: I was ready for bed.

Father to nurse: Then they did a little program. And they had a picture of her with her cast on sitting in bed.

Observer to parents: She's really making a little progress then, huh?

Father to all: This girl who comes to do her physical therapy at the house, see—she's from this Arthritic Association in Westport. [Father points out the different people who are in the picture.]

Nurse to child: You're really in the news, aren't you, huh? I didn't realize you were so important.

Mother to nurse: The people are lovely. We just go up there [referring to the Arthritis Association]. She [referring to the physical therapist] even bought her a half a gallon of ice cream.

Nurse to mother: Uhuh.

Mother to nurse: That encourages her. You'd be surprised what a little chow does.

Observer to mother: I'm not, I'm a nurse, but I'm not a pediatric nurse. But I'd say the parents and the children who I've seen here this past week while I've been doing this are just absolutely heroic.

Mother to observer: This place is wonderful.

Observer to mother (continuing): You know, both the strength and courage that those parents and children have to have.

Mother to observer: Right. I just spent five weeks with her here. You know, I stayed here like oh practically every day, for four or five hours. And the way they help one another. They really cooperate with you. Of course you're all discouraged and you're tired and you're travelling. The girls from high school will be playing with them.

Observer to mother: Really?

Father to all: Yes, they brought the school up to them.

Mother to all: Yes, they did, that was quite a thing. The photographer said, that should have gone in the paper. But, see, at the time, that's when I had the operation, I was just about standing up and he said—take her to the school. Couldn't even take myself. So you know what they said? "Is it alright if they take it there?" I had 35 kids at my house with all their boots and everything on. The boots were all covered with ice, but, I said let them enjoy it. She really loved it. She took all her guests up.

Nurse to mother: Isn't that nice?

Mother to nurse: Uhuh.

Father to nurse: She really came a long way, though, you know.

Nurse to father: Yes, I know.

Nurse to child: If you get better, honey, you won't have any publicity. [All laugh.]

Father to nurse: You don't want publicity that bad.

Nurse to parents: She's had enough? [All laugh.]

This passage points out the ability of this family to establish and maintain the initiative throughout the interaction. Although the nurse initially attempted to establish a medical orientation in terms of the child's weight problem, through the father's and mother's insistence the area of attention was shifted to the family's need for support in the home environment. This shift in focus was accomplished only by the persistent efforts of the father to direct the attention of the nurse to the write-ups about the child.

The initial response of the nurse to the father's introduction of pictures from the arthritis circular was to comment on how much heavier the child was at that time. The father disrupted this medical response by introducing another story with pictures from the arthritis association paper and the mother introduced a further write-up from the local newspaper, commenting with pride that it was carried in the lead column. Father and mother then introduced additional clippings moving the conversation away from medical issues and emphasizing the outside support they had received.[7]

As the observer was drawn into the conversation, the father and mother discussed with her the experiences of the family with the arthritis association, and its help to them in coping with the illness of the child. The mother also mentioned the encouragement they had received from the hospital during the daughter's recent stay there.[8] The supportive comments of the observer and the urgent demands of the family for attention to their home-related needs finally drew a response from the clinic nurse.[9] The comment, "If you get better, honey, you won't have any publicity," drew laughter from all present. This comment, judged from the relieved laughter of the family, provided the communication of support sought by the parents and their child during the interview.[10]

[7] The coalition between the parents in this family resembles the stable-supportive pattern identified by Strodtbeck in families and by Mills in three member task groups. Cf. Fred Strodtbeck, "The Family as a Three Person Group," *American Sociological Review,* XIX (February, 1954), pp. 23-29. Cf. also T. M. Mills, "The Coalition Pattern in Three Member Groups," *American Sociological Review,* XIX (Dec., 1954), pp. 657-667; and T. M. Mills, "Power Relations in Three Person Groups," *American Sociological Review,* XVIII (August, 1953), pp. 354-355.

[8] The relationships between father and mother in this family support Reiss' observation that the father may assume leadership *outside* the family, as in this case in confronting the hospital. However, the mother's leadership role in coping with the illness *inside* the family was clearly evident in this interaction. Cf. Ira L. Reiss, "Marital Roles and Small Group Research," in *The Family System in America,* New York: Holt, Rinehart and Winston, 1971.

[9] The contribution of the observer during this interaction and during that with several other families suggests Bruyn's and Gans' comments on avoidance of the "problems of over-rapport". The observer by volunteering support to the family, pointed up the problem of the clinic in dealing with emotional problems. During the second year, when observers did not manifest these tendencies toward "over-rapport", the arthritis clinic staff had initiated a policy of support which rendered these problems of "over-rapport" obsolete. The observers' change in behavior thus served to highlight alterations in clinic policy. The question remains whether observer influence had an effect on the alteration of clinic policy. The indications are that this effect was negligible. Cf. Severyn T. Bruyn, *The Human Perspective in Sociology: The Methodology of Participant Observation,* Englewood Cliffs, N. J.: Prentice-Hall, 1966, pp. 229 ff. Cf. also Herbert J. Gans, *Urban Villagers,* New York: Free Press of Glencoe, 1962, pp. 343-345.

[10] The heavy reliance of the nurse upon the observer before altering the original medical focus is consistent with Roth's assertion that a skilled occupation tries to keep the initiative in relation to the client. With the help of

II-9. Family Initiative and Home Scope

This interaction showed a dramatic shift in the area of discussion from a medical focus to the family's efforts to deal with the treatment and acceptance of the illness. By a series of interventions by the parents and the observer, emphasis was placed on the need for support for the child in coping with home problems. The nurse finally accepted the re-definition of the issue by providing encouragement to the family in its efforts toward adjusting socially to the disease.[11]

II-10. Patterns of Initiation and Scope of Problems

The pattern of interaction with this family illustrates a trend that existed throughout all the outpatient clinics. This was the tendency for families to talk about home-related issues, and for staff to discuss technical, medical problems. The tension that existed within the interview during discussion of activities in the home community clearly illustrates this tendency.[12]

The arthritis clinic in the first year manifested this conflict between family and staff perspectives more dramatically than any other service examined in the course of the research. When examination room interaction between families and staff is analyzed in terms of medical or technical scope of content, only 31.7% of the activity was initiated by families. On the other hand 68.4% of staff-family discussion involving home scope issues was family initiated. This sharp discrepancy in ex-

another health related person the nurse legitimized the change in the direction of conversation sought by the family. Cf. J. Roth, "The Treatment of Tuberculosis as a Bargaining Process," in A. Rose, ed., *Human Behavior and Social Processes,* Boston: Houghton Mifflin, 1962, pp. 575-588. The consultation with the observer also illustrates the unequal power distribution and plea bargaining which marked negotiations between health personnel and families. Cf. T. Scheff, "Negotiating Reality: Notes on Power in the Assessment of Responsibility," *Social Problems,* XVI (Summer, 1968), pp. 3-17. Cf. also M. Balint, *The Doctor, His Patient and the Illness,* New York: International Universities Press, 1957.

[11] The re-definition of the situation suggests the unstable accommodation between ecological givens and normative demands proposed by Rosengren and De Vault, "The Sociology of Time and Space in an Obstetrical Hospital," in Freidson, ed., *The Hospital in Modern Society,* p. 287.

[12] This tension parallels the incompatible expectations of hospital and family discussed by Bell and Zucker. Cf. Norman Bell and Robert Zucker, "Family-Hospital Relationships in a State Hospital Setting: A Structural Functional Analysis of the Hospitalization Process," *International Journal of Social Psychiatry,* XV (Jan., 1964), pp. 73-80.

amination room interaction as to medical and home scope issues was not equalled in the other outpatient services.[13]

The reasons for this contrast are well illustrated by the dynamics within this interview. Arthritis by its uncertainty and chronicity, inevitably poses many home problems. Familiarity with the clinic over long periods of time gave families a personal claim on the attention of physicians and nurses in seeking help for and recognition of these home issues.

Due to the lack of organization and planning there was a strong tendency for the staff not to respond readily to these home problems. Rather, they attempted to define difficulties in physical and medical terms. Only by persistent efforts, exerted with the social support of a health related network provided by the arthritis association could families obtain help from the staff on problems that were not directly medical.[14] The disparity between staff and family initiative in home related problems dramatically indicates the initial failure of the arthritis clinic to properly assist families with these non-physical issues.[15] However, almost as much activity took place at home scope as occurred at

[13] Cf. Appendix B, Table II, for percentages of staff and family initiation by scope during examination room contact in the various clinics.

[14] The role played by outside voluntary health networks in increasing the solidarity of families in bargaining with staff is consistent with Mills' analysis of the dominance of affective ties over values and manifest interactive patterns in small groups. In the present research, emotional attachments, when fortified by health association networks, were instrumental in overcoming differences in staff and family values and in altering prevailing interactive structures. Cf. T. M. Mills, "The Coalition Pattern in Three Member Groups," *American Sociological Review,* XIX (December, 1954), pp. 657-667. For related materials cf. T. M. Mills, "Power Relations in Three Person Groups," *American Sociological Review,* XVIII (August, 1953), pp. 351-357; T. Caplow, "A Theory of Coalitions in the Triad," *American Sociological Review,* XXI (August, 1956), pp. 489-493; G. Psathas and S. Stryker, "Bargaining Behavior and Orientations in Coalition Formation," *Sociometry,* XXVIII (June, 1965), pp. 124-144; R. De Charms, "Affiliation Motivation and Productivity in Small Groups," *Journal of Abnormal and Social Psychology,* LV (1957), pp. 222-226; W. A. Gamson, "A Theory of Coalition Formation," *American Sociological Review,* XXVI (June, 1961), pp. 373-382; R. H. Willis, "Coalitions in the Tetrad," *Sociometry,* XXV (December, 1962), pp. 358-376. [For a further discussion of coalitions as they relate to power relations in the present research, cf. V-8 (Chapter V, section 8.)]

[15] This disparity between family and staff initiatives, and the use of family networks as reference groups to obtain attention to home problems, illustrate a pattern of "co-orientation" consistent with Newcomb's "ABX Model". Cf. T. M. Newcomb, "An Approach to the Study of Communicative Acts," *Psychological Review,* LX (November, 1953), pp. 393-404.

medical scope, indicating the degree of family energy brought to bear on this staff resistance.[16]

II-11. Affective Patterns with Association Families

As shown by this father, mother and child, association families tended to dominate both in small talk (defined as diffused, non-goal oriented affective behavior) and courtship (defined as goal-directed affective behavior). Only after persistent efforts to entice the nurse in this direction was the family successful in changing the course of conversation.

This pattern of intense courtship was accompanied by generous amounts of friendly small talk. This behavior was typical of families belonging to voluntary health associations, not only in arthritis but also in the other clinics. These families came to the clinic with fairly well defined goals, and used active methods of appeal in prevailing upon the staff to obtain their objectives.[17]

Thus the pattern of interaction of association families was distinct from that displayed by other family units. Oriented to clear objectives, association families were more goal directed than were families not thoroughly familiar with arthritic medicine. Unaffiliated families usually took their cues during the course of conversation from the staff.[18]

II-12. Staff Support and Prior Hospital Contact

The handling of problems by families and staff was notably altered when, through prior contact, the problems to be discussed were already known to the clinic staff. Prior knowledge of family difficulties influenced the choice of problems dealt with and the approach taken to them.

[16] Cf. Appendix B, Table II, for frequencies and percent of initiation of home and medical scope in the arthritis clinic, especially during examination room interaction.

[17] This pursuit of self-directed goals by association families in relation to the staff illustrates the imbalance of institutional and opposition values discussed by Blau. Cf. P. M. Blau, *Exchange and Power in Social Life,* New York: John Wiley and Sons Inc., 1964.

[18] Families belonging to voluntary associations concerned with chronic illnesses illustrate both adherence to conduct rules (conformity) and investment in the ideology of the health organization (commitment). This commitment along with conformity to rules was effective in getting special attention from the staff. These families, especially in arthritis, exemplified the longitudinal and lateral biographical interest dimensions specified by Lefton and Rosengren for active client membership roles. Cf. M. Lefton and W. Rosengren, "Organizations and Clients: Lateral and Longitudinal Dimensions," *American Sociological Review,* XXXI (December, 1966), p. 806.

The influence of prior family contact on staff and family behavior is illustrated by an interview with a mother and a seven-year-old daughter. The interaction with this family commenced with the mother expressing her relief that the daughter had just been allowed to remove the braces required for her treatment. The response of the staff nurse to this family, who were known from earlier visits to the clinic, was quite decisive.

Mother to nurse: No more braces!

Nurse to mother: Oh, good. I wondered what you were all grinning about.

Mother to nurse (very excited): Yeah, no more braces! Just think of it! Almost two years . . .

Nurse to mother: Gosh, have they been on that long! [Several inaudible comments between family and nurse take place at this point.]

Nurse to mother: I'll never forget that day!

Mother to nurse: Oh that poor woman, now I feel bad for her.

Nurse to mother: I've never seen . . .

Mother to nurse: We had . . . the kids. Everybody was so upset! Oh, she had us real crazy! I'll never forget her!

Nurse to observer (explaining the situation): One of the other parents . . .

Mother (interrupting): Oh, it was terrible!

Nurse (continuing): . . . had Mrs. Godfrey rather upset, because she told her that the only reason you wear a brace like this is if you have a rotting hip. I hate to use the term.

Observer to nurse: A rotting hip, oh, my.

Mother (emphasizing nurse's story): That's what she said.

Nurse to observer: That was the day she was told to wear the brace.

Mother to observer: The first day we found out about it. Her two children had braces and we started talking. "Don't let her put that . . . it means a rotten hip." The brace is . . . then she said they'll replace it . . .

Nurse to mother: If I ever wanted to sock anybody in the nose, it was that woman. [They all laugh.]

Mother to nurse (first words inaudible): I couldn't talk. I was crying.

Nurse to mother: I don't blame you, you were really worried.

Mother to nurse: I was really worried.

At this point the nurse turned to the observer and explained some of the technical procedures in the care of the child's condition. The nurse cautioned the mother and daughter about the need to show special care during the initial period after the removal of the brace. The mother then spoke of her fears when the child was first put in the brace. She stressed her doubts about the physician who decided upon the child's treatment. The nurse expressed full understanding of the misgiving of the mother who in turn, later in the interview, expressed her acceptance of the correctness of the medical decision. The mother and child seemed to have been visibly relieved at having the opportunity to talk about their fears of the brace.

To some extent the contrast between the conversation with this family and that with the association family in the previous interview was due to the medical scope of the issues discussed. The nurse seemed more able to identify with the hospital-related problems of this mother and daughter, than with efforts of the earlier family to cope with the illness by means of the home arthritis association.

Since the nurse had shared the experiences of the second family, and because these experiences took place within the hospital, support was willingly provided. With the previous family, the observer assumed the initiative in providing reassurance which was finally picked up by the staff nurse. In supporting the second family in their feelings about wearing the braces, the arthritis nurse assumed the initiative and only relied upon the observer when tension mounted from specific anxiety-provoking issues.[19]

II-13. Small talk, Courtship and Prior Hospital Contact

The pattern of affective behavior with this mother and daughter about the problem of the braces, sharply contrasted with that involving the arthritis association family. The nurse responded immediately with support for the family's pleasure at the removal of the cast. She helped the mother and child recall their feelings when the cast was first put on. The anger expressed against the second mother for arousing fears about a "rotting hip" may be viewed as a courtship effort by the nurse to encourage the mother to express her earlier anxieties.

This courtship initiative was of help to the mother and daughter in expressing their apprehensions. The nurse also showed understanding of the mother's doubts about the wisdom of the physician who recommended the cast. This was also a courtship effort.

The success of the nurse in inducing this family to air its feelings illustrates the courtship pattern employed with families that were well

[19] There were a number of cases showing the tendency to deny support to families with social-psychological problems when neither external social networks nor internal hospital ties were available to them.

known from prior contact. The state of disorganization in the arthritis clinic precluded ordered interviews based on prepared study of clinic notes. Families attending the clinic needed special networks to obtain adequate health care. Such care was negotiable by families who carried on active courtship based on experience gained in the arthritis association. However, more ready attention was provided to families having friendly relations within the social network of the clinic. The role of the nurse as a key member in these internal hospital networks was a partial antidote to the disrupted care that marked the arthritis clinic during the first year.

II-14. Absence of Social Networks and Failure of Support

In a substantial number of cases families visiting the clinic had little previous experience with the hospital. This was the case for families with children who had recently diagnosed arthritis problems or who had just been referred to the hospital for treatment. These families lacked the social orientation available to those that have been discussed. Absence of previous contact with the clinic staff deprived uninitiated families of insider networks within the hospital.[20] Unfamiliarity and timidity in the clinic situation reduced their ability to bring to bear pressure on the staff in order to obtain special attention to their individual needs. As strangers to the hospital system, these families were not able to make use of their experience in outside social networks to take the lead during interviews with the staff.

The disorientation of families that lacked previous contact was exemplified by a conference involving a seven-year-old girl whose parents were under the impression that the child's colds were a cause of arthritic problems. The family voiced additional concern that stiffness in the joints might have been brought on by bicycle riding. They also expressed anxiety about the child's school problems.

No effort was made by the nurse to deal with the problems that this family was experiencing in accepting the illness and its social consequences. The family was told that colds merely aggravated the arthritis condition, and were directed to discuss the matter of bicycle riding with the physician.

The absence of health-related networks inside and outside the hospital deprived them of influence over the staff in gaining attention to their social and emotional needs. This family, and a number of others visiting the clinic, had not gained entry into these networks. Courtship by staff was minimal and unrelieved anxiety inhibited family small talk.

[20] Cf. W. F. Whyte, *Street Corner Society: The Social Structure of an Italian Slum,* Chicago: University of Chicago Press, 1955.

A significant number of families had not become members of arthritis social networks. This fact reduced the level of affective behavior in the clinic, and contributed to a marked structuring of the interactive roles of staff and family. These trends were partly attributable to the social disorganization in the clinic, but were most pronounced with families lacking health network ties.

II-15. Dependency Needs and Failure of Support

The examples cited of successful supportive nursing activity suggests that the needs of parents and children in arthritis were of a dependency variety. Families needed encouragement in their efforts to normalize the lives of children handicapped with chronic disabilities. They needed to have their fears of casts allayed and their anxieties about doctors' judgments reduced. Families who had strong ties through the arthritis association or through personal contacts in the hospital, were able to negotiate support for these dependency needs. They sought and obtained the reassurance of the staff in their efforts to help their children put up with the uncertainties of the illness. However, a number of families who lacked appropriate health networks were not able to negotiate the terms of the satisfaction of their dependency needs. Their isolation resulted in the failure of the support of dependency needs in the old arthritis clinic.

II-16. Quantitative Analysis: Arthritis Clinic as a Staff Based Improvising Organization

A computer analysis of coded data derived from the transcribed tape recordings has been developed with a view toward making a quantitative analysis of the clinic as a staff-based improvising organization. The analysis of the computerized data indicates the strong tendency of the nursing staff to use medical areas for contact with families. Thus virtually all interaction (97%) involving nursing personnel and families took place in the examination rooms. This compared with lower figures for examination room contact with families in the other outpatient services (83% in orthopedic, 35% in diabetes, and 8% in cystic fibrosis).[21]

An improvising pattern of interaction is characterized by a relatively high degree of family initiative; an emphasis on home and life cycle issues rather than technical medical ones; a fairly free and open form of emotional expression; and a rather relaxed structuring of interactive roles. On the other hand, sharp role structure, affective restraint, staff initiative and medical scope are characteristics of ritual interaction, a pattern particularly evident in the cystic fibrosis clinic. (For ritualized

[21] Cf. Appendix B, Table Ib.

elements in the latter clinic, see below, Chapter VIII-22. Cf. also Appendix A, Methodology, A-5 and A-6, for discussion of the empirical dimensions of improvising and ritual interaction.)

The prevalence of family initiative during examination room interviews underscored the designation of the clinic as a staff-based improvising institution. A substantial proportion of staff-family interaction (44.3%) was originated by families, the highest such percentage recorded during the research.[22]

The tendency for families to assume the initiative is also substantiated by a computer analysis of the scope of problem content dealt with during staff-family interaction. Thus in the arthritis clinic medical scope issues constituted a minority of interaction content (45%), with substantial attention devoted to home scope (38%) and life-cycle scope (17%) problems. In contrast, the majority of problem content was devoted to medical issues in cystic fibrosis (89%). Predominant attention was also given to medical scope problems during diabetic (87%) and orthopedic family interaction (67%).[23]

These patterns of emphasis on home and life cycle problems in arthritis are substantiated by further analysis of the data. A lagged regression analysis statistically isolates the effect, over a period of time, of one variable upon another after eliminating the influence of all other variable factors.

This statistical isolation procedure, when interaction in the clinic was analyzed sequentially on an act-by-act basis, showed that home and life cycle issues had a remarkable stability over time.[24] Only in arthritis did home and life cycle issues maintain this high level of continuity along with medical scope problems.

The great stability of interactive content is clearly shown in Graph A-II-16 which compares patterns of interaction over time in the arthritis and orthopedic clinics. The graph indicates that—over an average span of four interactions in arthritis—medical, home and life cycle issues remained remarkably stable. Over the same span, and at each step in the process, all three types of issues were notably less stable in the orthopedic clinic.

[22] This compared with 28.5% in diabetes, 36.4% in cystic fibrosis and 36.7% in orthopedics. Cf. Appendix B, Table II.

[23] Cf. Appendix B, Table Ib.

[24] Thus after the fourth step of interaction a high correlation (0.708) was shown for maintenance of home scope issues. (Cf. Appendix B, Table III.) A similarly high level correlation (0.658) was maintained for life cycle scope problems over four steps of interactive process. The fact that medical scope problems also maintained constancy (0.670) over this interactive span points to the remarkable stability of issues discussed over time in the clinic. (Cf. Appendix B, Table III.)

GRAPH A-II-16

Stability of Scope of Content over Varying Numbers of Intervening Acts during the First Year

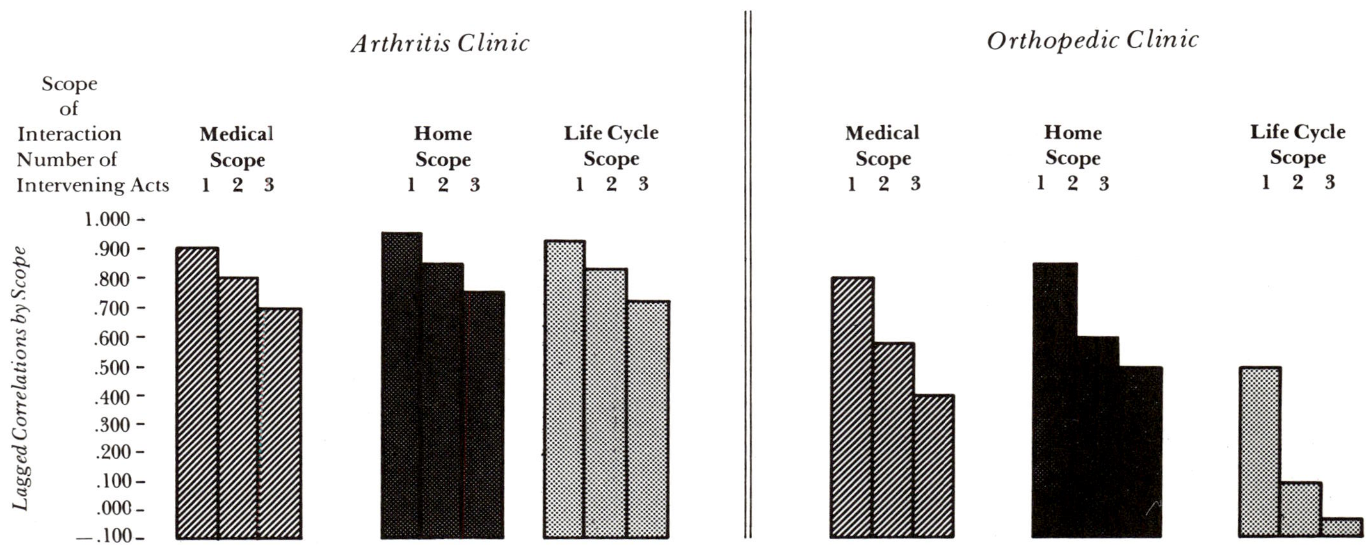

The above analysis is based on lagged correlations. cf. Methodology, Appendix, **A-6-***1, p. 199, for discussion of the use of lagged correlations.*

The stability of the scope of issues through the interactive process was a mark of the arthritis clinic as an improvising interactive system. Families, by virtue of their active role in interaction, were able to engage staff in sustained discussion of specific topics over extended periods. In the other clinics, where staff control was the rule, the scope of interaction tended to vary in accordance with the choice of physicians and nurses. Greater continuity of scope in arthritis was related to more intense engagement in the communication process through joint staff-family participation. The arthritis clinic thus presented several striking features of a staff-based improvising system.

II-17. Discordant Improvisation: Affective Restraint

Five types of emotional expression emerged from the interactive patterns generated by the various out-patient services. These affective patterns are isolation, suppression, restraint, chanelling and diffusion. In the course of the research the different clinics showed marked contrasts in affective patterning, while some services displayed pronounced shifts over time from one emotional interactive type to another.

Owing to the state of disorganization that originally prevailed in the arthritis clinic, a tone of affective restraint characterized the interaction of staff and families. This emotional inhibition was traced to the lack of planning for family interviews and the resultant reluctance of staff to provide emotional support to parents and children. Curtailment of feelings was also reflected in the hesitance of some families in pursuing discussion of problems with staff, a hesitance that was overcome only by thorough orientation to health networks inside and outside the hospital.

The inhibition of staff-family interaction in arthritis was revealed by an analysis of the affective variables, *small-talk* and *courtship*. The term *small talk* denotes emotional expression of a friendly or spontaneous sort viewed apart from any immediate practical objective. *Small talk* characterizes the positive feeling tone of the interaction apart from any other action-related context. *Courtship,* on the other hand, is emotionally charged behavior which is directed to a deliberate goal, typically involving collaboration with other parties.

A measure of affective process has been developed based on differences between relative levels of *reserved* and *expressed* feelings. *Reserved affect* is manifested by high levels of small talk and courtship put forth during periods of low work activity. This is interpreted as an affective reservoir of the interactive network. *Expressed affect* is indicated by high intensities of small talk and courtship exhibited during phases of very active work activities.[25]

[25] Reserved and expressed affective ratios are derived by dividing the frequencies of these two types of intense emotional behavior by the frequency of

Based on the relative difference between expressed and reserved feelings different affective patterns of interaction may be distinguished. A sharp preponderance of expression over reserve indicates diffusion, while a moderately high expressive imbalance suggests affective channelling. A slight positive bias in favor of expression manifests emotional restraint, while the predominance of reserve over expression indicates affective suppression and isolation. Affective diffusion and channelling are associated with improvising networks; and restraint, suppression and isolation of feelings suggest ritualized interaction.[26]

Three of these affective patterns were evidenced by the various clinics during the first year. Thus as shown in Graph B-II-17, the arthritis and cystic fibrosis clinics displayed patterns of affective restraint. In both these services there was a slight tendency for feelings to rise in intensity during heavier work periods, relative to rest sequences. Both clinics were marked by moderate overall feeling levels.

On the other hand, in diabetes feelings rose dramatically during phases of intensive work, while remaining *relatively* low during less work-oriented activities. This pattern was one of diffused feelings.

In orthopedics a contrasting model of isolation of feelings was evident. Emotions rose during periods of social rest but fell rather noticeably during work activities.

In arthritis, a cross tabulation analysis of small talk with courtship,[27] and of courtship with feedback opportunity and service activities revealed a moderately high expressed affect[28] which was narrowly in excess of reserved feelings.[29] The small positive expressive balance[30] suggested a pattern of affective restraint. Feelings which were at all times fairly closely held in check, were only slightly increased with more intensive work activities.

The affective restraint that marked interaction in the arthritis clinic related to the organizational constraints which were operative during the first year of the research. Under-staffing and unplanned family interviews put the staff under heavy pressure to avoid intimate contact with parents and children, as indicated by minimum levels of staff initiated feelings.[31] Similarly, because of staff resistance to friendly

all low intensity feelings manifested during social interaction. Cf. Methodology, Appendix A, Section A-6-3, on the concept of affectivity.

[26] For more complete discussion of affective behavior, cf. Appendix A, Section A-6-3.

[27] Cf. Appendix A, Section A-6-3, fn. 14, for discussion of courtship as both an affective and a task oriented variable.

[28] With a ratio of 1.001; Appendix B, Table VII, Col. 4.

[29] Indicated by a ratio of 0.782; Appendix B, Table VII, Col. 3.

[30] +0.219; Appendix B, Table VII, Col. 5.

[31] Staff courtship was at a level of 2.140, whereas staff small talk showed a mean of 2.298. Cf. Appendix B, Table XVIII.

GRAPH B-II-17

Patterns of Affective Behavior in the Four Out-Patient Clinics during the First Year

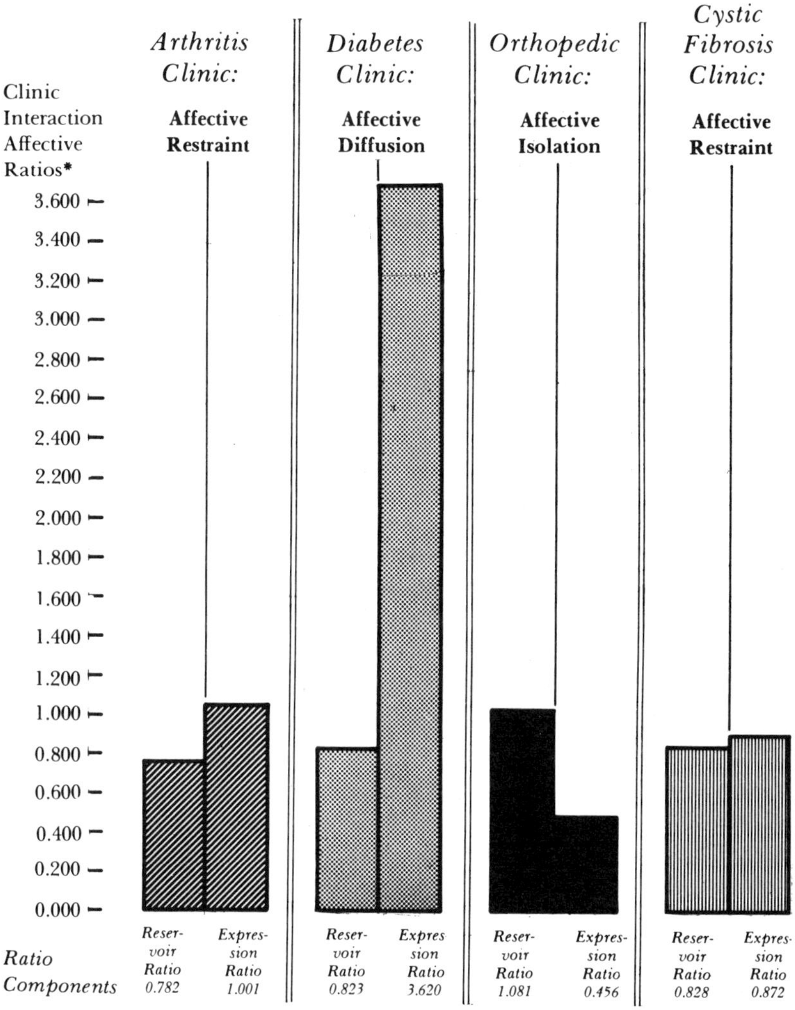

Procedures for deriving the reservoir and expression ratios are described in the methodology.* **Appendix A-6-3*, p. 199 under the concept of affectivity. Cf. Appendix B, Table VII, Cols. 3 & 4, for ratio values.*

approaches, family courtship and small talk were also withdrawn. Thus the expressive dimension, conceptually associated with an improvising pattern of social interaction, was restricted in the dynamics of affective restraint as indicated by the cross-tabulation analysis.

II-18. Sharp Differentiation of Roles

In a sharply differentiated system, staff assumes role dominance in courtship and in creating opportunity for feedback, establishing a pattern of rigid and directive leadership. In contrast family members dominate in small talk and in providing feedback in a correspondingly passive and submissive pattern. Strict structuring of roles was particularly notable in ritualized services such as the cystic fibrosis clinic.

However, in the first year's operation of the arthritis services a similarly rigid pattern was observed. The tendency for staff to trail behind families in the expression of small talk was due to desire to avoid close contact with families.[32] This withholding of small talk was matched by family reticence in courtship.[33]

Even more dramatic differences, however, took place in task behavior. A relatively high intensity in providing feedback was shown by families in contrast to the staff.[34] In effect responses to inquiries were virtually all provided by families.[35] Similarly in providing opportunity for feedback, staff dominated over families.[36] This provided a composite picture of staff inquiries, with families passively providing needed information. Despite the activity displayed by families in overall initiating patterns, specialized feedback behavior betrayed the

[32] Family initiated small talk showed a mean of 2.970, whereas the staff level was only 2.298. (This difference accounted for an ETA value of 10.3% in regard to this latter variable.) Cf. Appendix B, Table XVIII.

[33] Thus family initiated courtship showed only a mean of 1.804 as compared with a family initiated small talk mean of 2.970. Cf. Appendix B, Table XVIII.

[34] As reflected by a family mean of 1.658 and a staff mean of 1.038. Cf. Appendix B, Table XVIII. In arthritis, scores for all variables relating to staff-family interaction were based on 199 "bits" of family initiated activity, and 235 staff-initiated interactive "bits". The determination of a "bit" of interaction was based on a complete thought or sentence, consistent with the method of interaction process analysis. All means are based on a coded rating scale of one to five, with the number *one* assigned to zero intensity of the activity, and *five* to maximum intensity. Cf. R. F. Bales, *Interaction Process Analysis,* Cambridge: Addison-Wesley Press, 1951. Cf. Appendix A, Section A-4, for a discussion of scaling and coding procedures.

[35] This family dominance accounted for an ETA value of 11.2%.

[36] With a mean of 1.860 as compared with a family mean of 1.226. Cf. Appendix B, Table XVIII.

strong need for staff control and the incapacity of families to take command of the communication process.[37]

The fact that greater disparities in family and staff initiative occurred in arthritis than in the large bureaucratic setting of the orthopedic department, points to the rigidities that marked the arthritis services during the first period of the study.

The overall pattern in the clinic was one, therefore, of staff control of goal-directed behavior matched by a general family passivity. The result was a quite structured system, a discordant pattern for an improvising interactive system.

Despite strong overall family initiative and prevalence of home-related issues, the clinic presented some features of a ritualized (i.e. a structured and restrained) interactive system. These features were related to the organizational problems of the clinic. Because of the degree of family initiative and the emphasis on home related problems a potential existed for a more dynamic interactive system. This potential was effectively exploited in conjunction with organizational factors which came into play with the move of the arthritis services to the new outpatient building.

II-19. Discordant Improvisation and Weak Feedback Responsiveness

The presence of discordant elements in the arthritis clinic viewed as an improvising interactive system was associated with poor performance during feedback processes especially by families. Failure of responsiveness was indicated by an act-by-act or sequential analysis of family feedback measured against immediately preceding acts involving opportunity for feedback. Thus family initiated feedback only increased slightly (by 6.7%) in response to previous efforts to obtain information. This compared with a greater intensity (of 35.3%) on the part of staff members in providing feedback following attempts to procure information.[38] This discrepancy suggests that families were singularly sluggish in participating in the feedback exchange.

[37] These figures, based on analysis of means, are supported by an analysis of correlations for family initiation as compared with staff initiated activities related to the feedback process. The correlation analysis reveals that families dominated in the intiation of feedback and small talk, while staff controlled courtship. Opportunity for feedback, while negatively correlated for both, was much less likely to be initiated by the family than by staff members. (Cf. Appendix B, Tables IV and V; medical scope problems are presented in the correlations to permit comparability statistically with the other clinics.)

Overall difference in correlations between staff and families on the four feedback-related variables produced a higher total divergence (1.296) than was noted in the orthopedic clinic (0.911).

[38] Cf. Appendix B, Table VI.

The feeble contribution of families to the feedback process in arthritis is brought out by comparison with the orthopedic clinic. Thus as shown in Graph C-II-19, orthopedic families were slightly more dominant than staff in a moderately high overall 25.2% average feedback response. In arthritis, however, staff sharply dominated a low overall response pattern that only averaged 16.0% in staff-family feedback sensitivity. While a balanced pattern of exchange prevailed in orthopedics, a communication gap marked the apathetic feedback in arthritis.

The low rate of family responsiveness to requests for feedback is closely associated in arthritis with the affective inhibition and the weak connection between courtship and opportunity for feedback. Family reticence during the feedback process was also connected with the rigid role structure that characterized the clinic's functioning in the old building. Although families provided notably higher intensities of feedback than staff,[39] family feedback was not part of an ongoing mutual process. Families simply assumed the role of passive purveyors of information to be judged or acted upon by the staff.

Excessive information-seeking by the staff was a related phenomenon. The dominance of staff inquiry had an anaesthetizing effect upon families in providing information. A glut of questions, inhibition of feelings, sharp role differences were serious interactive defects in the old arthritis clinic viewed as a staff-based improvising system. These defects seriously hindered the ability of the clinic to cope in a sensitive manner with the long range issues of families with arthritic children.

The sharp contrast between family concern with home problems and staff focus on medical issues indicated the failure of the clinic to support parents' efforts to care for their children in the home community. Families with special network resources were able to negotiate support for these efforts. Overall, however, the arthritis clinic failed to provide support for the dependency needs of families.

[39] Shown by a feedback mean of 1.658 as compared with 1.038 by the staff. Cf. Appendix B, Table XVIII (with an ETA value of 11.2% for the difference).

GRAPH C-II-19

Feedback Responsiveness by Families and Staff in the Arthritis and Orthopedic Clinics during the First Year*

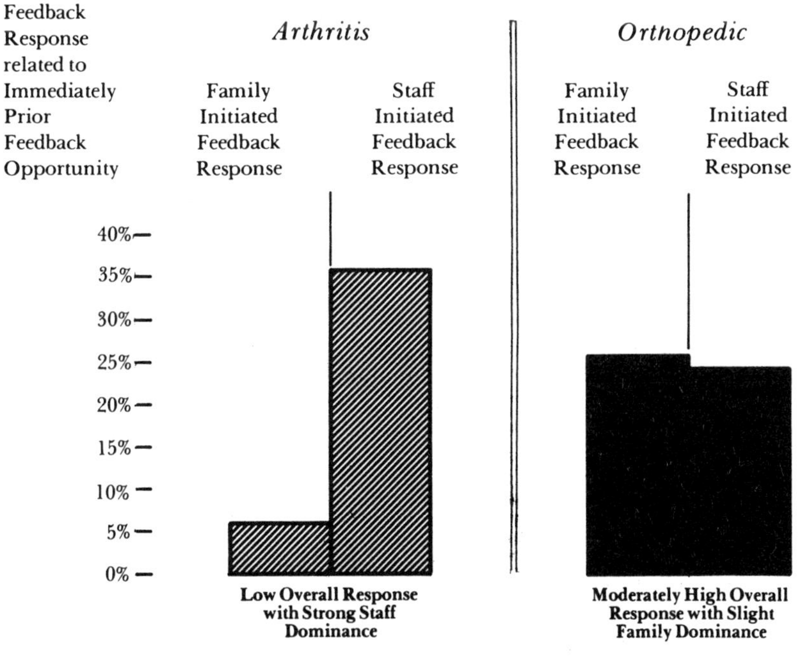

Arthritis	*Orthopedic*
Average (unweighted) Family-Staff Feedback Response=16.0%	*Average (unweighted) Family-Staff Feedback Response = 25.2%*
Specific Feedback Response	*Specific Feedback Response*
Family=6.7%	*Family=26.2%*
Staff=35.3%	*Staff=24.2%*

Based on lagged regression analysis of data presented in Appendix B, Table VI, p. 207. Cf. Appendix* **A-6 *p. 199 for related discussion of the concepts of structuring and responsiveness.*

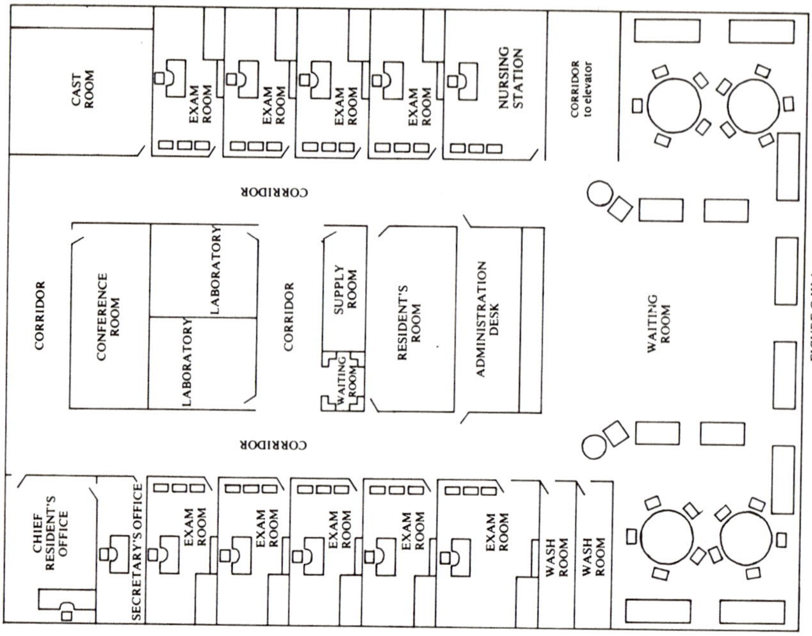

FIGURE C-III-1
DIAGRAM OF A TYPICAL OUT-PATIENT CLINIC DURING THE SECOND YEAR

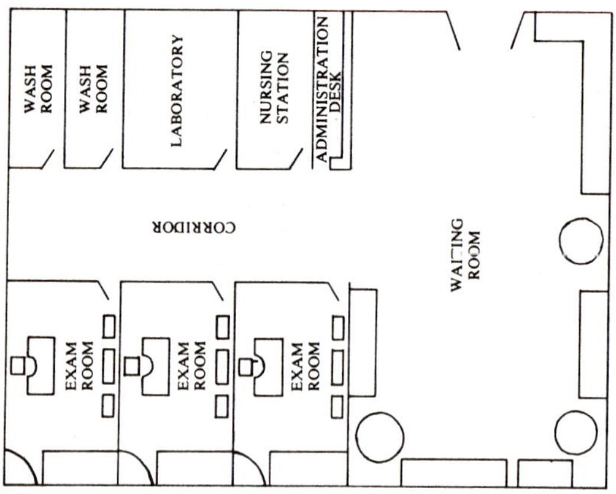

FIGURE B-III-1
DIAGRAM OF A TYPICAL OUT-PATIENT CLINIC DURING THE FIRST YEAR

CHAPTER III

THE ARTHRITIS CLINIC: CHANGE IN A STAFF BASED IMPROVISING ORGANIZATION

The beneficial change in the delivery of health services to families brought about by the relocation of the arthritis clinic was unique among the outpatient services. The clinic though politically powerful, lacked effective medical control; a discrepancy which contributed, in the new setting, to its further evolution as a staff-based improvising institution.

III-1. Factors Affecting Change in the Arthritis Clinic

Along with the physical and personnel changes that accompanied the move of the outpatient clinics to the new building, certain organizational factors produced specific trends in the delivery of arthritis health services. Compared with the other clinics, the arthritis department was a considerably smaller unit, with an average of four or five families seen during a clinic session.

Several important organizational changes accompanied the move. During the first year some families with arthritic children were contacted in the general orthopedic clinic. In the new building two sessions of two hours each week were set aside to provide for the health needs of all arthritis families. This arrangement made it possible for families to meet with the staff in relatively quiet conditions, removed from the confusion of the general surgical services. Much longer periods of staff time were devoted to families who had to face the complex problems posed by the illness.[1]

Moreover, prior to the move to the new facilities the nursing department had made some important policy decisions. Arthritis is a complicated illness which requires of health personnel considerable knowledge of its dynamics. Its unpredictability makes planning of family interviews very difficult.

The nursing department adopted a clinic nursing specialist approach. Although the same senior nursing personnel were retained, intensive effort was made to educate the staff to the issues and problems confronting families. A prominent change occurred in the ability of the nursing staff to respond in the course of interviews. As clinic nursing specialists they became more sensitive to family efforts to deal with the range of problems provoked by the illness.[2]

A number of physical and organizational factors contributed to an upgrading of arthritis health services. Among these was an increase in the number of examination rooms available for family contact. Replacing the three rooms of the orthopedic clinic, six examination rooms were reserved for the exclusive use of arthritis families. A new clinic clerk was responsible for administrative details, while a nursing assistant was provided to the staff nurse to take care of routine medical tasks. There was an increase in medical staff, so that the constant irritation of absences and shortages of physicians, which marked the old location, was reduced. Moreover, a new senior resident was placed in charge of medical operations, resulting in improved performance by physicians. (See Figure C-III-1 for a general diagram of the new clinic facilities.)

III-2. Changes in Staff Relations

These physical and organizational changes, along with the policy shifts that accompanied them, led to modifications in staff relations.

[1] Time spent in staff-family interaction increased from 57.5% to 78.0% in the second year. This compared with declines of 62.0% to 43.8% in cystic fibrosis, 64.6% to 55.1% in diabetic, and 43.6% to 41.7% in orthopedic. Cf. Appendix B, Table X.

[2] The education of staff entailed in developing this new nursing specialist policy suggests an *anticipatory* and *innovative* approach to change as stipulated by Lowthrop. The policy of the clinic manifested a "reaction to detected forces of change before they emerge in overt and dynamic form" which specifies "*anticipatory* and *innovative* . . . . adaptation to change." Cf. L. C. Lowthrop "The Environment, Bureaucracy and Social Change," in A. Bartlett and T. Kayser, eds., *Changing Organizational Behavior*, Englewood Cliffs, N. J.: Prentice-Hall, Inc., 1973, pp. 19 ff.

During the first year staff members criticized the organization of the arthritis services. The clinic during that period suffered from weak medical leadership and a shortage of physicians, nurses and clerical personnel. These problems were reflected in administrative difficulties. Reduction of nursing entanglement in administration at the new location was reflected by a noticeable decline in contact with subordinate clerical staff (shown by the shrinkage of such interaction from 25.0% to 16.8%).

A marked change also occurred in relations between nursing staff and physicians. During the first year a substantial portion of nursing time (17.6%) was spent attending physicians during examinations and interviews with families, or in providing technical assistance to doctors. In the new clinic, time devoted to these subordinate medical tasks declined sharply (to 5.2%). Moreover, a significant portion of this reduced contact with physicians resulted from the initiative of nurses who obtained specific medical services that had been requested by family members.[3]

III-3. Changes in Staff-Family Relationships

During the previous year 57.5% of clinic time involving the nursing staff had been occupied with actual contact with families, while the remaining 42.5% was taken up with staff matters. This low rate of encounter was due to the administrative problems.

In the new outpatient building, with the reorganization of arthritis services, 78.0% of clinic time involving nurses was spent in direct contact with families, while staff activities declined to 22.0%. No other service of the outpatient department showed such a sharp increase in the attention given to families. In fact the other clinics each declined in rates of family contact.[4]

The increase in the percentage of arthritis staff time devoted to consultation with families was parallelled by a marked growth in absolute time spent with families. The average time for family conferences expanded from 16½ minutes to 54 minutes, a more than threefold increase.

[3] The success of the nursing service in obtaining these family requests from physicians supports Mechanic's observation that when lower participants become more influential in complex organizations high ranking members become more dependent upon them. Cf. D. Mechanic, "Sources of Power of Lower Participants in Complex Organizations," *Administrative Science Quarterly* VII (December, 1962), p. 349. For shifts in nursing interaction with physicians and staff, cf. Appendix B, Table X.

[4] Cystic fibrosis declined in staff-family contact by 18.5%, diabetes by 9.5% and orthopedic by 1.9%. Cf. Appendix B, Table X.

III-4. Use of Ancillary Clinic Personnel

While the availability of additional examination rooms was vital, uninterrupted lengthy family contacts were also facilitated by the presence of ancillary nursing and clerical staff who assumed routine clinic duties. On a number of occasions with the help of these new members of the clinic staff it was possible for the nurse to continue an interview in the examination room, which might earlier have been disrupted. This constructive use of ancillary personnel distinguished arthritis from all of the other outpatient clinics during the second year.[5]

III-5. The Examination Room as Staff Based Care Center

In some of the outpatient clinics a separate care center emerged where staff instruction in the autonomous handling of treatment was carried out. In diabetes the waiting room developed as a care center apart from the examination rooms, where cure functions were carried on. Similar practices were followed in the cystic fibrosis clinic.

In arthritis, because of uncertainties and unpredictable changes, delegation of responsibility to the family was not emphasized. The need was for an authoritative stance on the part of the clinic staff. The strategy of the staff, and particularly of the head nurse, accented the management of dependency. The nurse in the face of family uncertainty and anxiety (reflected at times in her own awkwardness) presented herself as an authoritative representative of the staff physicians. A medical image was projected by the nurse during extended and unbroken family contacts in the examination room. Her goal was the reduction of family anxiety by building confidence in the efficacy and competence of arthritic medicine.[6]

The use of the examination rooms as a care center to achieve this goal was indicated by the fact that 78% of all staff-family contact was

[5] This assistance from ancillary personnel confirms the view of Mechanic that informal coalitions arise in place, tasks only being fully coordinated at high levels in complex organizations. The head nurse's use of charismatic qualities as a senior person in the arthritis department is also consistent with Mechanic's contention that lower participants employ attractiveness to establish access to control over persons. Cf. D. Mechanic, "Sources of Power of Lower Participants in Complex Organizations," *Administrative Science Quarterly*, VII (December, 1962), p. 349. The fact that in arthritis administrative problems were staff-related, made possible the delegation of the tasks to subordinates. In the orthopedic clinic where families themselves were constantly embroiled in obtaining scarce services from the hospital, delegation of these responsibilities to ancillary personnel was not effective.

[6] The access of nursing personnel to the examination rooms for extended contact with arthritis families accords with the position of the head nurse as a

conducted in that area. Although this was a decline in arthritis clinic practice from that of the previous year (97%), only the orthopedic clinic (with 79%) surpassed arthritis in examination room contact.[7] Moreover, family examination room contacts were far more lengthy in arthritis than in any of the other clinics.

III-6. Example of Staff Based Family Contact

An example of the use of the examination room as a care center devoted to the management of dependency, is provided by a nursing interview with a mother and her fifteen-year-old son. The adolescent boy was suffering from rheumatoid arthritis, complicated by an epileptic condition. The mother, who displayed extreme anxiety, had recently changed the aspirin dosage without obtaining the permission of the physician. She felt guilty, fearing the side-effects of excess aspirin. She also expressed concern about the long-run effects of arthritis on the life pattern of the child.

Having discussed the limited nature of side effects of aspirin, the nurse attempted to quiet the family's fears and build their confidence:

> **Nurse to mother:** And, this is a strange thing about arthritis, that— that there aren't very many chronic diseases in—known to— a—to medicine that can be handled by something that seems as simple as an aspirin. But, an aspirin is not a simple thing at all. My grandfather used to say . . . it was the smartest pill around because it always knew where to go to find the ache. I suppose he was right. Aspirin is a very valuable drug. The other two things are rest and immobilization. Um.
>
> **Mother to nurse** *(while she is talking):* Yes, I know about that.
>
> **Nurse to mother:** And casts or something like that.
>
> **Mother to nurse:** Oh!
> [*She seems surprised.*]
>
> **Nurse to patient:** Or on crutches. And, should your knees—a—have an attack, probably, the doctor would put on crutches for a while. Or, have you get in bed for a little while. The problem he had with your [sic] heart was the most severe thing that can happen. The business you are having with your finger now is not unusual.

"boundary-spanning" "discretionary" person (Thompson) within an institutionally discrepant unit of the hospital. Cf. below, III-15, nursing opportunity for this power access. Cf. D. Mechanic, "Sources of Power of Lower Participants in Complex Organizations," *Administrative Science Quarterly,* VII (December, 1962), p. 319. Cf. also James D. Thompson, *Organizations in Action.*

[7] Cf. Appendix B, Table Ib.

Mother to nurse: No! he said it's gone. He said, Wednesday, because [he] said it was Ash Wednesday.

[Observer's Comment: In the conversation above it is difficult to tell where the nurse is talking to the patient and where she is talking to the mother. On several occasions the mother has answered where it was definitely the patient to whom the nurse was speaking. Just above, I thought she was speaking to the mother and that she had not used personal pronouns for some time but that she then used "you" in the way that sounded like she was addressing the patient. This mother seems to be dominating the conversation. She seems quite defensive and in some ways over-protective. She does not seem to be acting as one would expect the mother of a 15-year-old child to act.]

Nurse to mother: This weather erases [symptoms], you know.

Mother to nurse: Ya. But no. He hasn't complained though. Because, I thought, in the beginning, you'd hear all the old times and me, I wasn't there even. [*She laughs, referring apparently to "old age" arthritis.*]

Nurse to mother: Ya.

Mother to nurse: Because, you know, well, you say, "Gee, if they have pains!" But, he doesn't.

Nurse to mother: Well, ya. The old timers. It's an old age kind of arthritis which [is] a little different from this, too.

Mother to nurse: Oh.

Nurse to mother: Kind of an old rheumatism.

Mother to nurse: Um. [*Pause.*] So, this is actually different from the regular rheuma [tism] . . .

Nurse to mother: This is . . .

Mother to nurse: Rheumatism?

Nurse to mother: This is . . ., this [is] different [from] that rheumatism. This [is different] than the arthritis that comes on you when you're sixty years. . . . sixty years old. This is a little bit different and needs to be handled a little bit differently. And, it . . . a . . . it is something you can live with. But, when you say that you don't have to sound so down about it . . . because it doesn't have to interfere with your life . . . with your life. [*The nurse's last few comments seem to be directed to the patient.*] And, of course, when it hurts you, you'll know it. And when it doesn't hurt you, you'll forget you had it.

Mother to nurse: Well, that's what he does! Yes!

Nurse to mother: Sure.

Initially the nurse attempted to build confidence in the power of aspirin to handle the pain associated with arthritis. This was done by resorting to folklore. Aspirin was dramatized both for its simplicity and for its magical ability to find the area of pain. The nurse appealed to the experience of her relatives as testimony to aspirin as a pain reliever.

The use of magical and folk[8] allusions is of interest in the management of dependency. The comments were made in the context of arthritis as a chronic disease. The family was consoled with the thought that the disease could not be too severe if its pain could be controlled by such a simple cure. By implication, the family should not fear the side-effects of aspirin since generations have known of its beneficent effects.

The nurse also reviewed the procedures for dealing with the physical complications of the illness. In addition to aspirin, rest and immobilization might be prescribed. The description of these procedures was accompanied by the attempt to assure the mother that the young boy, within limits, might expect to have a normal life.

III-7. Reliance on Medicine and Over-Protectiveness

The observer commented that the mother appeared to be dominating and over-protective toward the adolescent boy and defensive toward the nurse.

The defensiveness was related to her guilt at having changed the dosage without the physician's approval. The guilt was due to the serious illness of the child who had suffered from various ailments since infancy. The over-protectiveness of the mother seemed to represent an attempt to compensate for this prolonged poor health.

The nurse responded to this over-protectiveness with an effort to build confidence in arthritic medicine. Although no claim was made for a cure of the condition, its various symptoms were described as ameliorable. Thus, with usual degrees of pain aspirin was advised; if discomfort should increase various types of rest and immobilization were recommended. The nurse proposed the protection and authority of arthritic medicine as a relief for the anxiety and guilt of the family.

Although it is not clear that the nurse was successful in establishing this confidence in medicine, this was the intent of the strategy pursued. This became more evident at the end of the interview when the mother inquired about the possibility of a dietary cure for arthritis. The nurse squarely denounced such claims as the advice of quacks. This denunciation was received by the mother with some chagrin.

Although the nurse was probably not successful in establishing full

[8] Cf. Jerome David Frank, *Persuasion and Healing, A Comparative Study of Psychotherapy*, Baltimore: Johns Hopkins Press, 1961.

confidence in the arthritis staff, it is clear that the intent of the rhetoric was to establish unwavering trust.[9]

III-8. Management of Dependency and Acceptance of the Illness

The approach taken with this mother and fifteen-year-old son was lacking in sensitivity. The nurse appeared overwhelmed by the anxiety of the family, and seemed to be merely authoritative rather than sympathetic.

A contrast was provided by the case of a mother and her four-year-old daughter. This family was much more prepared to deal with the emotional issues posed by the child's illness, which was not so complicated as that of the previous family. The mother of this young girl was very much upset at not having been told earlier of the severity and probable long-term nature of the child's disease. She also complained that the illness had been discussed by physicians in front of the child, which had been upsetting to the daughter.

The comments of the mother and the response of the nurse took place in the examination room of the clinic:

Mother to nurse: . . . Right now, I can't help but think if I had been told what to look for, I might have seen it even sooner and you might have been able to get her in the hospital even sooner for treatment and maybe even all of the traction she would have missed. I just feel that I'm uninformed.

Nurse to mother: I'm trying to do that to a point now. Right now, things are changing and when I get a definite diagnosis which may mean a long time . . . month, a year, then sit down and to talk about the potentials of the future. The fact that winters are going to be different than summers and school may be different for the child and these things which are going to come up. Even the possibility of getting a stomach ache from aspirin. There is only so far that I can go because I'm not the doctor. And every mother has to be handled individually. Some can only swallow one thing at a time—others like it set out for them . . . and this is . . . of course you

[9] The apparent failure to instill trust during this interview may be analyzed in terms of Lewin's concept of "steering" as a feedback method for evaluating action. There was ample evidence during this interview of the "discrepancy" between "desired and actual progress," which should have led to "corrective change". The "discrepancy" rose from the anxiety of the mother which prevented her from absorbing the advice offered by the nurse. "Corrective change" might have suggested more efforts at emotional support to deal with the underlying anxiety. Cf. K. Lewin, "Feedback Problems of Social Diagnosis and Action" in W. Buckley, ed., *Modern Systems Research for the Behavioral Scientist: A Sourcebook,* p. 441.

can't walk into a room, and say now do you want me to tell you everything at once.

[Observer's comment: Mother laughs freely. Most of the nervousness has disappeared from her face and from her voice; it seems that she is at ease.]

Nurse to mother: I have to use, what I can, upstairs. I think in your case that if you make it clear to anyone of the doctors, of course, you get a change of doctor . . .

Mother to nurse: Ya, that's true, too. That gets a little annoying too.

Nurse to mother: You make it clear to them and to the nurses should she be admitted and it's not inconceivable that she might have to be admitted another time for the same thing. Right in the beginning, that you've run up against these things and you have been disappointed and you would like to know, in as much as possible, how long term. That you don't want these things mentioned in front of Charlotte. No, do it! Because there are some teenage situations in particular where we can't say a word in front of the kids. Otherwise, the mother can't, you know, they accuse the mother . . .

Mother to nurse: Well, I was, really . . . hard because they kept her in here, anyway. Because it was the last thing I expected.

Nurse to mother: That was not expected. No. No, that was not expected.

Mother to nurse: No, I came up here just for a check up and everything got thrown for a loop at that point, you know.

Nurse to mother: I think they wanted her in for more than traction too.

Although the nurse was sympathetic to the mother's complaints, the support was couched in terms of deference to physicians on the staff. The nurse prefaced her comments by stating that she was "not a doctor" and any information she would give the mother would have to depend upon a definite diagnosis by the physicians. The nurse also hedged her comments by pointing to the hesitance of hospital staff "to tell you everything at once."[10]

Having built her defenses in relation to the staff, the nurse counselled the mother to demand from physicians her right to be told about her child's condition. She then conceded that the physicians had pre-

[10] This hesitance illustrates Sussman's finding of the lack of staff appreciation of outpatient families' need for knowledge of the illness. Cf. M. B. Sussman et al., *The Walking Patient: A Study in Out-Patient Care,* Cleveland: The Press of Western Reserve University, 1967, p. 130.

viously admitted the child for reasons beyond the expressed need to change treatment procedures.

While encouraging the mother to demand her right to be told about the child's condition, the nurse urged her to insist that the illness not be discussed in front of the child. The effectiveness of the nurse's counsel on these delicate issues may be judged by the fact that the mother proceeded to bring up two more problems of greater urgency which were bothering her.

As the conversation continued the mother touched on whole new areas:

Mother to nurse: . . . There's this idea. She is due to go to school. In September, now I, it dawned on me a little while ago that I'd better not be telling this child all along you're going to school regardless. Because I don't know what's going to come up. But it took me a while to really realize this. You know, there's a little girl down the street the same age who will be going to school in September. Now I find out this month that we really don't know what's going to happen with this, and rather than get her all built up to the fact that she's going to be going to school next September . . .

Nurse to mother: Oh, that's rough. Because they look forward to school.

Mother to nurse: Ya, I know, but this is the thing that I had to figure out for myself. No one warned me "don't be telling her she's going to be going to school." Well, I saw a little boy up here and talked with a mother who thought he was going to go to school in September and found out now that he isn't. You know, and the first thing you say to kids when you meet them at that age is, you know, "Are you going to school?" or "When are you going into school?"

Nurse to mother: She might be, you know.

Mother to nurse: And he just . . . oh, you know . . .

Nurse to mother: They're not going to know till August.

Mother to nurse: Oh, I know that. I realize that. But the thing is I don't want to get her all built up. Because she's going to go on that school bus with the other kids in the neighborhood, and these are different things which, you know, you kind of have to go by . . . [The mother's words are covered by a page on the PA system.]

[Observer's wording is bracketed in the following passage when the mother's or nurse's speech was inaudible.]

Mother to nurse: And I wonder if there is any way the parents can be helped [in the very special handling of the children because they're certainly not going to have the average life. The same as the other kids].

Nurse to mother: And yet, we won't—we want more than ever to have these kids treated as normally as possible—and on . . .

Mother to nurse: Yes, and that's the problem trying to treat them normally when they're [inaudible word]. [*Laughter.*]

Nurse to mother: I know it. It's such a delicate balance between overprotecting and . . . a . . . you see, of course, I see it swing both ways. I see youngsters that aren't allowed out of the house . . . out of mother's reach, and I see others who hurt . . . who are pushed.

Mother to nurse: Um, so that's a hard thing to do yourself when you're dealing with therapy or something like that. You are not too surè just how far to go sometimes.

Nurse to mother: Ya, it just takes knowing your own child.

Mother to nurse: Yes, somedays you go like crazy, you know, and another one of these things is the traction, it's getting very, very difficult.

During the latter phase of this interview, the mother and nurse showed a more mutual relationship in discussing the child's school problems. A rapport had been built (facilitated by the removal of the child from the examination room by a nursing aide), which enabled the nurse to communicate understanding and feeling for the mother's anxiety about the education of the child.[11]

[11] The emphasis on rapport and understanding during the first portion of this interview is congruous with Thompson's description of "heuristic-optional transactions." Thus in the early stages of interaction, a large portion of behavior of both parties is oriented toward establishment of rapport and a small proportion, toward the content of the "transaction relationship." The concentration on past problems of a more diffuse nature before tackling the immediate issues facing the family toward the end of the interview is consistent with this emphasis on building of rapport. Cf. J. D. Thompson, "Organizations and Output Transactions," *American Journal of Sociology*, LXVIII (November, 1962), p. 320. The sensitive treatment of the problems of this family appears to take account of the factors stimulating effective two-way communication regarding psycho-social issues as articulated by Zola. These include the importance of privacy, adequate time for staff-patient interviews and appropriate contact with personnel other than physicians. Cf. I. Zola, "Problems of Communication, Diagnosis and Patient Care: The Interplay of Patient, Physician and Clinic Organization," *Journal of Medical Education*, XXXVIII (October, 1963), pp. 829-838.

Also the nurse showed sensitivity in offering advice to help the child lead a more normal life. Extremes of over-protection and of too heavy demands on the child were pointed out. Toward the close of this sequence when the mother confided "you are not too sure how far to go sometimes," she appeared to be conveying her trust and confidence in the understanding of the nurse.

This confidence was rewarded when the mother brought up the problems that the child was experiencing in sleeping with the traction devices prescribed by the clinic. After a brief description of the problem by the mother, the nurse excused herself and quickly arranged with the physicians for the equipment to be changed so the child could sleep more comfortably.[12] Having received new instructions from the nurse, the mother left the examination room, her anxieties for the child greatly relieved.[13]

III-9. Staff Based Care Functions and Acceptance of the Illness

According to the comments of the observer, this mother was on the verge of tears at various points during this interview. At the end of the interview, when the emotional and technical problems of the family had been thoroughly discussed, the observer, commenting on the nurse's sensitivity in dealing with the needs of this family, indicated that the mother left the clinic "much happier."[14]

The ability of the nurse to provide emotional and technical assis-

[12] Families exploited "strains" in the system presented by nursing occupancy of medical areas to elaborate a more effective delivery of services from the hospital. Cf. Buckley on the role of normal strains in system elaboration, *Sociology and Modern Systems Theory,* p. 130. The active approach adopted by arthritis families where the uncertainity of the illness made planning of interviews difficult suggests Dill's analysis of the bargaining behavior of customers when they were not ordering standard products. Cf. W. Dill, "Environment as an Influence on Managerial Autonomy," in *Administrative Science Quarterly,* Vol. II (March, 1958), pp. 521-541.

[13] This sequence of interaction also suggests the characteristics of effective feedback as specified by Deutsch. These include a communications network which produces action in response to an input of information and includes the result of its own action in the new information by which it modifies its subsequent behavior. K. W. Deutsch, "Toward a Cybernetic Model of Man and Society," in W. Buckley, ed., *Modern Systems Research for the Behavioral Scientist: A Sourcebook,* Chicago: Aldine Press, 1968, pp. 387-400.

[14] Although a relatively low status person within the hospital hierarchy, the nurse as a health professional had sufficient position relative to this family to provide important and satisfying support. Cf. related comments by N. H. Berkowitz and W. G. Bennis, "Interaction Patterns in Formal Service-Oriented Organizations," *Administrative Science Quarterly,* VI (June, 1961), pp. 25-50.

tance to this family was remarkable when compared with the behavior of the staff during the first year. This change in the quality of health service was underlined during the interview by the assistance of the nursing aide who removed the child from the examination room at the request of the nurse. This intervention enabled the contact to continue for about an hour. It is also interesting that the delicate emotional problems relating to the mother's acceptance of the child's illness were brought up only after the removal of the child. (The parallel here with the previous family suggests that the presence of the child might have inhibited discussion of touchy issues.)

Supported by the nurse, the mother was able to express her irritation at not being told about the gravity and long-range character of the child's condition.[15] Having introduced these enduring problems, and having received sympathetic understanding from the nurse, the mother was prepared to bring up more immediate and pressing difficulties. Among these were the school problems of the child and her difficulties in sleeping with the prescribed traction devices.

Only when the nurse insisted in firm tones on the mother's right to demand from the physicians an explanation of the nature of the child's condition did she present her immediate worries.

The underlying difficulty of this family was acceptance of the illness. The physicians were not prepared to tell the mother of the long-range character of the illness because they were not sure of her ability to cope with this problem. The nurse, by insisting on the mother's right to an explanation, affirmed confidence in her ability to cope with it.

This confidence was reinforced by the support given to the mother's plea that the illness not be discussed in the child's presence. The nurse expressed her solidarity with the mother in having to face the distress of the child. The mother was more able to accept the child's long-term illness if she did not at the same time have to deal with the additional fears of the daughter. It was the understanding which the nurse brought to the mother's need to cope with these long-range issues that was the key to the quality of this interview. When the long-range issues of acceptance of the illness had been discussed, the mother was prepared to deal with the short-run issues of school and mechanical sleeping arrangements.[16]

[15] The mother's irritation about having the illness discussed in front of the child was closely related to the need of the mother herself to be told about the nature of the illness.

[16] The prior settlement of these long-range problems before the bringing up of immediate pressing difficulties is related to Mills' observation of the initial "intimacy issue" faced by groups prior to effective task engagement. In the case of coping systems, families may resolve the intimacy issue with staff by

The ability of the nurse to provide effective assistance to this family in coping with the long-range problems of arthritis was made possible by continuous, extended and undisturbed occupancy of the cure center of the clinic. In the examination room the nurse carried out care functions with an assurance and status derived from the cure activities of the physicians.[17]

The nurse supported this mother's need to accept the illness by assuming the medical manner of management of dependency. For a subordinate person such as a nurse to assume such authority toward physicians required the backing of the medical setting of the examination room.[18] For care functions to take on an aggressive stance in the cure dominated atmosphere of the hospital required extended occupancy of the cure center by the nurse. Backed by the medical authority of the examination room the nurse was able to combine assurance with sensitivity in assisting this family to accept and cope with the illness.[19]

III-10. Support of Dependence and Acceptance

The interaction between the nurse and this family illustrates successful

introducing more remote life issues as a way of judging the degree of support staff can provide for more urgent matters. Cf. T. M. Mills, "The Coalition Pattern in Three Member Groups," *American Sociological Review,* XIX (December, 1954), pp. 657-667. The efforts of the nurse to secure the acceptance of the illness by the mother through supporting her demands on the physicians suggests Buckley's model of authority, cooperation and consensus. It is in contrast with the compliance and power structure approach found in the orthopedic clinic. Cf. W. Buckley, *Sociology and Modern Systems Theory,* pp. 176-186.

[17] The decrease in strain evident in the nursing assumption of greater authority during examination room interaction in the new clinic can be understood as a successful fulfillment of system demands through "role bargaining" in accordance with Goode's analysis. Cf. W. J. Goode, "A Theory of Role Strain," *American Sociological Review,* XXV (August, 1960), pp. 483-496.

[18] By using a consensual approach the nursing staff attempted to routinize the charismatic authority of surgery. To the extent to which magical and folklore elements accompanied nursing interaction the charismatic quality of the authority remained. This pattern may be subsumed under the role of "charismatic follower" (suggested by Virginia Olesen in a personal communication). Cf. *From Max Weber: Essays in Sociology,* trans., ed. H. Gerth and C. W. Mills, New York: Oxford University Press, 1958, pp. 262 ff. For a more complete discussion of types of power and authority cf. W. Buckley, *Sociology and Modern Systems Theory,* pp. 191-205.

[19] This combination of authority and sensitivity is somewhat similar to the relaxing of affective neutrality by staff in the delivery room as reported by Rosengren and De Vault, "The Sociology of Time and Space in an Obstetrical Hospital," in Eliot Freidson, ed., *The Hospital in Modern Society.*

support in coping with the problems of chronic pediatric arthritis. The authority of the nurse, sustained by lengthy, unbroken contact in the examination room was important in establishing this mother's confidence in the hospital. The evident fears of the mother centered around her feeling that she had not been dealt with honestly or openly by physicians. The directness and sympathetic understanding of the nurse were effective in the mother's willingness to confide her feelings about her problems.

This confidence and dependency on the nurse elicited the mother's admission that the fears centered on the long-term uncertainties of her daughter's illness. These feelings were mixed with anger and frustration at the failure of physicians to be candid with her. The forthrightness of the nurse in insisting that the mother demand fair treatment from the doctors, served to calm her anger and ease her frustrations. The aggressiveness of the nurse therefore provided appropriate support to the mother in dealing with the hospital bureaucracy. The mother also received additional strength from the nurse in meeting the immediate problems facing the child. Thus the mother seemed more prepared to accept the uncertainties about the child's entry into school. Her willingness to depend upon the nurse for advice coincided with evidence of greater ability to accept the uncertainties of the disease. The successful support provided to this family was evidenced by this increase of trust and of willingness to face the issues.

III-11. Improvising Interaction and Decreased Structuring

In all of the clinics a general pattern of interactive specialization was noted in types of behavior emphasized by families and staff members. Based on computer analysis of numerically coded variables,[20] families tended to manifest high levels of diffuse affective behavior, in the form of small talk. Families also usually provided more articulate responses to inquiries, designated as feedback. Staff, on the other hand, specialized in more directive forms of affect, in the form of courtship; they tended to provide opportunity for feedback to families by opening up opportunities for them to provide information about their children. The tendency to specialize in these categories of activity had been quite pronounced in the old arthritis clinic, which was a sharply structured interactive network.

Increased continuity and sensitivity of communication between staff and families accompanied the organizational changes in the new arthritis services. An indication of the general upgrading of staff-family conferences was the decline in the rigid differentiation that had pre-

[20] Cf. Appendix A for a discussion of the coding and analysis of variables.

viously marked the interactive network of the clinic.[21] The decrease in differences between family and staff initiated small talk was especially prominent.[22]

Family initiated courtship increased, relative to that of staff, while staff opportunity for feedback declined relative to that initiated by family members.[23] None of the other clinics showed such a steep decline in role patterning in the course of the restructuring of the outpatient services. This striking shift toward destructuring of roles in the clinic suggested the emergence of the arthritis services as a fully developed improvising interactive system.

III-12. Destructuring and Improvisation

A sequential analysis of the interaction supports the trends toward a decline in differences of clinic roles.[24]As shown in Graph D-III-12, the pattern of typical role structuring expected of families and staff became notably less rigid. The reduced overall differences in correlations indicated the most flexible patterning of interactive roles observed in the course of the research. It is also worthy of note that the new clinic was unique as to family initiative in providing opportunity for feedback. In all the other research settings staff dominated in providing openings for

[21] This finding is consistent with that of Sussman showing that time spent with staff other than physicians is an important determinant of patient satisfaction. Cf. M. B. Sussman *et al., The Walking Patient,* p. 64.

[22] Thus a discrepancy of 0.672 in the mean of family over staff small talk was reduced to 0.245. Cf. Appendix B, Table XVIII. (The ETA value also declined from 10.3% to 1.7%.) A comparably sharp reduction was noted in the imbalance of feedback provided by families and by staff. Thus a family predominance in providing of feedback diminished from 0.620 to a figure of 0.155. (This decline resulted in a decrease in the ETA value for this difference from 11.2% to 1.6%.) Cf. Appendix B, Table XVIII.

[23] Cf. Appendix B, Table XVIII.

[24] Thus the total difference in lagged correlations during the first research period was 1.296. Total difference declined by 39.7% (to 0.782) in the new arthritis clinic. This degree of dedifferentiation of role activity was not approached at any time by the other outpatient services. Cf. Appendix B, Tables IV and V. As explained in the methodology, differences in role structuring are based on expected divergences in uniform role patterning, with families positive on small talk and feedback, and staff expected to be positive on courtship and opportunity for feedback. Cf. Appendix A, Methodology, A-6-1, *Structuring.* This marked reduction in role structuring approached the partnership model of patient care proposed by Szasz and Hollander more closely than any of the other outpatient services. Cf. T. Szasz and M. Hollander, "A Contribution to the Philosophy of Medicine," *A.M.A. Archives of Internal Medicine,* Vol. 97, No. 5, (May, 1956), p. 585.

the initiation of feedback processes. The dominance of feedback opportunity by families is further indication of the advance of improvisation as a characteristic of the clinic interactive network.

GRAPH D-III-12

Changes in Role Structuring* in the Arthritis Clinic
(medical scope interaction)

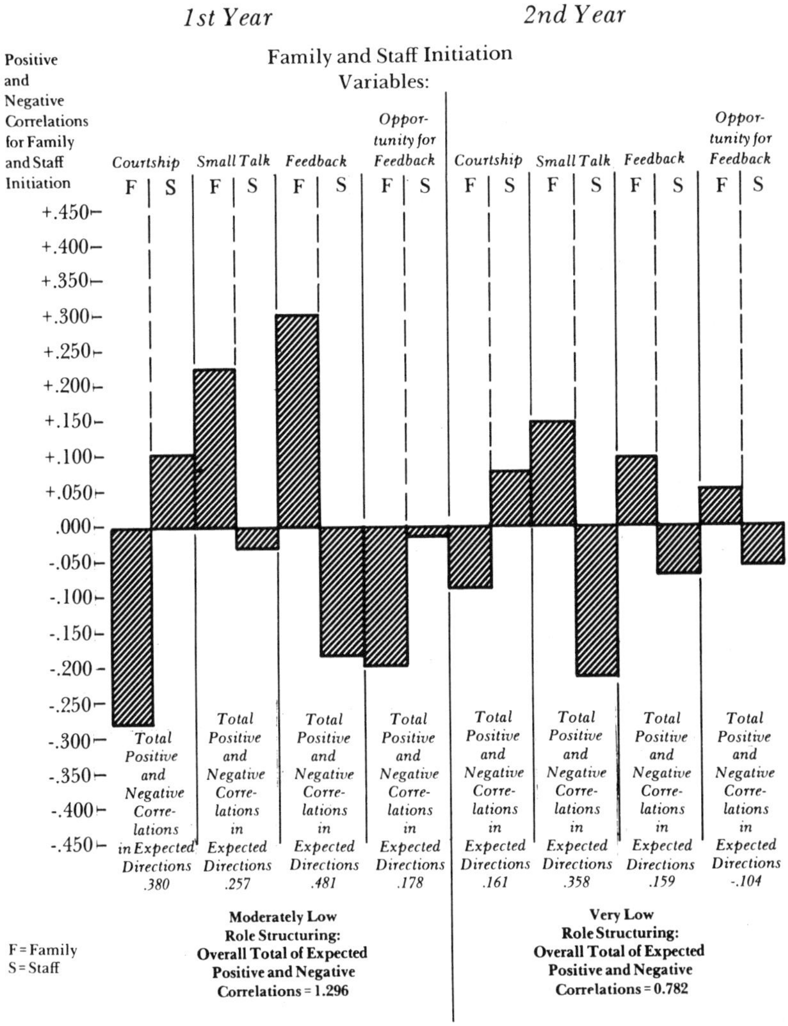

**Role structuring is based on expected family initiated positive correlations in small talk and feedback; and expected staff initiated positive correlations in courtship and opportunity for feedback. Negative correlations are expected for family initiation of courtship and opportunity for feedback, and staff negative correlations are expected for small talk and feedback. The analysis is based on lagged correlations presented in Table IV, Appendix B, p. 204.*

III-13. Affective Restraint and Channelling

It has been noted that during the first period of the research a pattern of affective restraint characterized the interaction in the arthritis clinic. Feelings in the clinic were largely held in check due to the state of organizational disarray associated with understaffing, crowded facilities and ineffective leadership. Despite the ability of individual families to elicit support from staff due to unique health network advantages, the overall behavioral profile was one of social distance and inhibition.[25]

With the move some notable changes occurred in the expression of feelings during staff-family interaction. This shift indicated a movement from restraint to affective channelling as a system characteristic.[26]

The changes in affective behavior in the clinic are shown in Graph E-III-13. An increase in expressive dominance along with a moderate rise in the general level of feelings indicated the emergence of channelling as the emotional pattern of clinic interaction.

In a qualitative sense, interaction during work-related sequence was characterized by a moderately high intensity of positive feeling, and feelings tended to rise perceptibly during task-oriented passages, and to decline somewhat during non-work connected interaction. The picture of social exchange in the clinic was, therefore, of a system in which feelings were employed in a directed positive manner during work activities, while at the same time a modest but significant reservoir of feelings was preserved for non-work related matters. As a supportive system, the new arthritis clinic presented a model of interactive feelings available for working relationships, while retaining sufficient reserves of positive emotions for occasions of social respite. The directed character of feelings expressed when applied to work situations, combined with emotional resources maintained for socially de-

[25] These trends were reflected quantitatively in a moderately low overall level of affect (of 0.892) and a weak positive balance (+ 0.219) of expressed over reserved feelings during the conduct of goal-related matters, indicating a pattern of affective restraint.

[26] While reserved feelings during non-work related passages remained virtually on a par (with a mean ratio of 0.795 representing an upward increment of only 0.013) expressed feelings put in play during task-related activities increased notably (from 1.001 to 1.777 on the Expression Ratio). Cf. Appendix B, Table VII, Cols. 3 and 4. Thus the level of affective behavior rose in intensity from 0.892 to 1.286 based on a combined mean for work-related and non-work related feelings, (col. 6); while positive balance of expression over reserve showed a substantial increment (from +0.219 to +0.982). Cf. Appendix B, Table VII, Col. 5.

GRAPH E-III-13

Change in Components of Affective Behavior in the Arthritis Clinic

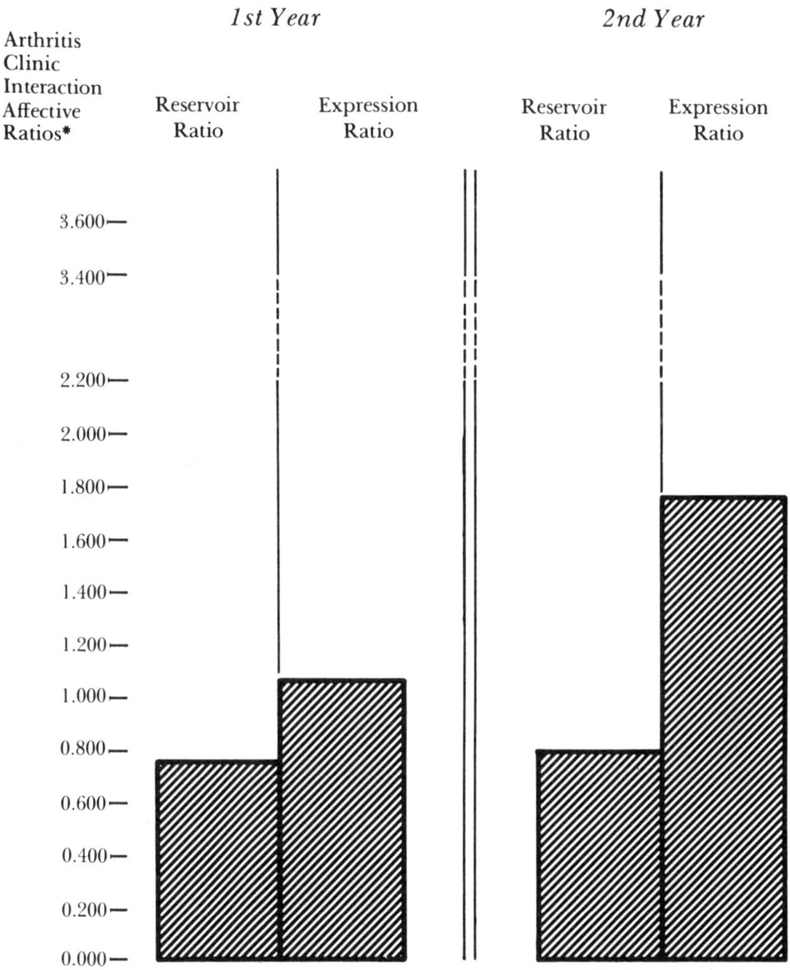

Affective Restraint: Weak Expression Dominance with Moderate Levels of Feeling		**Affective Channeling Moderate Expression Dominance with Moderate Levels of Feeling**	
Reservoir Ratio 0.782	*Expression Ratio 1.001*	*Reservoir Ratio 0.795*	*Expression Ratio 1.777*

* *Based on ratios presented in Table VII, Appendix B, p. 207.*

fined contexts pointed up the channelling of emotions in the clinic.[27] This affective channelling represented a positive trend in the arthritis services as an improvising support system coping with the problems of children and families attending the clinic.[28]

III-14. Affective Channelling and Feedback Responsiveness

Accompanying the shift from restraint to affective channelling in arthritis was an increased feedback responsiveness in the clinic. Thus while affective behavior was augmented during task activities, and emotional reserves were kept at a moderate high for socially defined situations, responsiveness during feedback activities became much more sensitive.[29]

Families had been faced with a glut of information seeking in the old clinic. High intensities of opportunity for feedback were initiated by staff, and correspondingly intense feedback was provided by families. However, feedback as offered by families was not in response to prior seeking of information, as shown by a variance of only 6.7% in response to feedback opportunity.[30] Families volunteered information

[27] This pattern of intensified feelings during work, and moderately high emotional tone during rest appears to reverse the trend observed in task oriented groups as reported by Bales. Thus groups tend either to be concerned primarily with problems of social integration, expressed by strong positive group feelings, or to be involved with external demands of the task, accompanied by lower positive emotional expression. The fact that the problems discussed are "internal" to the family, which uses the staff to gain support in coping with issues, may account for the absence of these polar trends in arthritis. Cf. R. F. Bales "Adaptive and Integrative Changes as Sources of Strains in Social Systems," in A. P. Hare, E. F. Borgatta and R. F. Bales, eds., *Small Groups: Studies in Social Interaction,* New York: Alfred Knopf, 1965.

[28] This pattern of affective channelling is consistent with the third order purpose of "preservation of process" ascribed to feedback communication networks by Deutch. Thus a moderate rise in feelings is devoted to immediate work on the task, while somewhat lower levels are reserved for less intense goal activities. These reserved feelings are available for work on future task processes and are also preserved for the well-being of the group or system. Cf. K. W. Deutsch, "Toward a Cybernetic Model of Man and Society," in W. Buckley, ed., *Modern Systems Research for the Behavioral Scientist: A Source Book,* Chicago: Aldine Press, 1968, pp. 387-400.

[29] The finding of Postner, of positive associations between "affective expression" and "good outcome" in family therapy, seems related to trends toward affective channelling in the arthritis clinic. Cf. R. S. Postner *et al.,* "Process and Outcome in Conjoint Family Therapy," *Family Process,* X (December, 1971), pp. 451-473.

[30] Cf. Appendix B, Table VI.

not as a result of an interactive process but consequent upon a tacit and rigid role assignment. Families provided information whether or not such communication was solicited. In many cases families provided information, especially about home situations, which was actively resisted by the staff.

In the new arthritis clinic a different type of interactive network came into existence. This was partially indicated by the reduction in structuring of interactive roles. Staff provided almost as much feedback as families, and staff were hardly more active than families in seeking feedback.

GRAPH F-III-14

Change in Feedback Responsiveness by Families and Staff in the Arthritis Clinic*

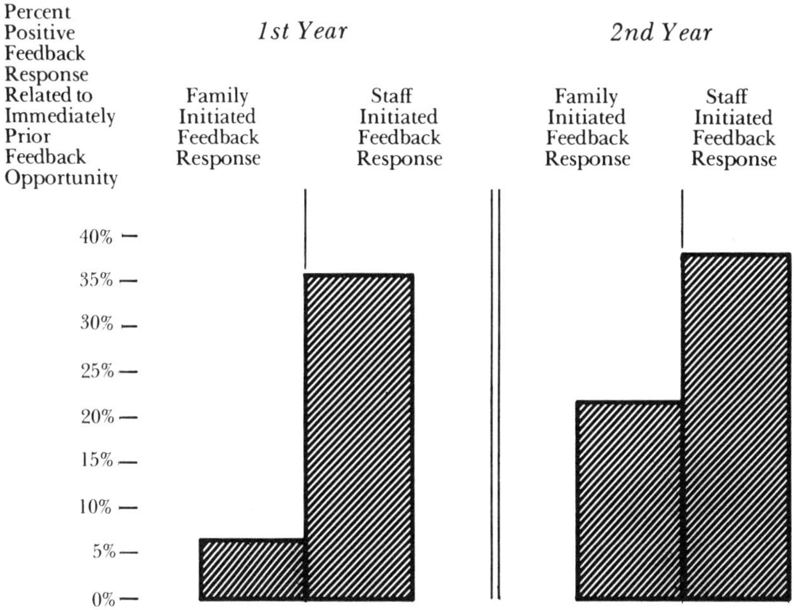

Moderately Low Overall Response with Strong Staff Dominance	**Moderately High Overall Response with Moderate Staff Dominance**
Average (unweighted) Family-Staff Feedback Response=21.0%	*Average (unweighted) Family-Staff Feedback Response=29.4%*
Specific Feedback Response:	*Specific Feedback Response*
Family=6.7%	*Family=21.0%*
Staff=35.3%	*Staff=37.8%*

**Based on lagged regression analysis of data presented in Appendix B, Table VI, p. 207.*

The increased reciprocity between families and staff during the feedback process may be seen in Graph F-III-14, which shows the reduction of the communication gap from the previous year.

The channelling of energies made possible a less busy feedback process (indicated by sharp declines in family feedback and staff feedback opportunity). Thus, in combination with the destructuring of roles, emotional channelling produced a more effective feedback responsiveness, as shown by a sharp increase in family response (from 6.7% to 21.0%). This steep rise was accompanied by a slight gain (of 2.5% to 37.8%) by the staff in responding to feedback requests. This resulted in almost the highest average family-staff feedback response (29.4%) observed in the outpatient service.[31] While quantity of information decreased, willingness to provide information when it was sought increased. This rise in responsiveness was particularly strong on the part of families, but staff also maintained a level of responsiveness that was higher than that attained in any other clinic. With an increase in affect channelling and decreased role structuring, the quality of the feedback process was upgraded as displayed by staff and family willingness to engage in reciprocal exchange of information.[32]

Increases in channelled feelings, when accompanied by role destructuring resulted in increases in effective goal-directed activity as indicated by more sensitive feedback processes.

III-15. Institutional Discrepancy and Increased Improvisation

In the case of arthritis a condition of high political power, derived from affiliation with the surgical departments, joined with an uncertain though ameliorative technology. With the move to the new outpatient quarters, the political power of arthritis became enhanced by greater nursing access to examination room facilities and nursing control over new clinic personnel. Owing to weak medical control, physicians yielded to nurses' access to these facilities and to their control over the services of ancillary staff in maintaining extended contact with families.[33]

Institutional discrepancy coupled with the weak technology and uncertainty of the illness also provided opportunity for initiative by fam-

[31] Except in the cystic fibrosis clinic with an unweighted average feedback response of 29.9%. Cf. Appendix B, Table VI.

[32] These qualities of communication in the new arthritis clinic are closely conformed to the elements of adaptive process as specified by Buckley. Cf. Buckley, *Sociology and Modern Systems Theory*, pp. 205-207.

[33] Institutional discrepancy thus plays a role in social decision making through dehierarchizing access to institutional resources. Cf. Buckley, *Sociology and Modern Systems Theory,* pp. 82 ff.

ilies. Parents employed new extended interviews with nurses as an opportunity for expressing demands on the hospital. Nurses in liaison with families were able to exert influence over physicians because of readier access to medical areas.[34] Availability of the power location of the examination rooms enhanced the authority and security of nurses resulting in greater sensitivity to family needs. The improved quality of staff-family interaction was reflected in the greater staff initiative toward home related issues. The significance of these trends was reflected in improvements in feedback responsiveness, especially on the part of families. In effect the exploitation of institutional discrepancy led to increased improvising interaction, which was marked by greater effectiveness in feedback functioning.[35]

The increase in sensitivity of communication as measured by feedback responsiveness is linked to changes in the clinic as a staff-based improvising institution. Longer contact in the examination room, emphasis on home scope problems and high level family initiative led to role destructuring and sensitive expression of feelings.[36] The qualita-

[34] This liaison between families and nursing in obtaining services from physicians is reminiscent of the "negotiated order" of the hospital discussed by Strauss. Cf. A. Strauss *et al.*, "The Hospital and its Negotiated Order," in *The Hospital in Modern Society,* E. Freidson, ed., New York: Free Press of Glencoe, Inc., 1963, p. 148. The behavior of arthritis families in these liaison activities with nurses, may be compared with the Cyert and March analysis of coalitions including active stockholders. Such stockholders become "*internal* members of the coalition," joining with management officials in determining policy. Thus arthritis families by the "aggressiveness" of their "bargaining" became "internal members" of the clinic, whereas orthopedic families, for instance, remained "passive" or "external members". Cf. R. Cyert and J. G. March, *A Behavioral Theory of the Firm,* Englewood Cliffs, N. J.: Prentice-Hall, Inc., 1963, especially, pp. 28-32. Cf. also footnote 3 in Chapter X for a related discussion of institutional discrepancies based on Perrow's analysis of technology as a factor in decision-making (p. 183, below).

[35] The interconnection between authority, security and sensitivity to needs points to positive connections between "spatial environment functions" as suggested by Steel. "Growth" occurs if a "spatial environment" stimulates people to "see similarities and differences in one another." Such "growth" conditions characterized longer examination room conferences in the new arthritis clinic. Cf. F. I. Steel, *Physical Settings and Organization Development,* Reading, Mass.: Addison-Wesley Publishing Company, 1973, especially, pp. 96-98; and pp. 4-22.

[36] The close interconnection temporally between affective and feedback components suggests Thompson's analysis of processes during "heuristic-optional transactions." Thus "each successive time the relationship is . . . challenged by the unfolding of information which bears on costs and rewards, rapport must be reestablished." This instability of relationships in respect to

tive analysis of family-staff interviews, suggesting an upgrading of the support of family needs for trust and acceptance of the illness, is consistant with the systematic quantitative analysis of the coded data. These observations in combination indicate the evolution of the clinic as a staff-based improvising institution[37] for coping with the problems of arthritis families.

threat from task activities suggests the imbalance toward affective needs which characterized interaction in the arthritis clinic. Cf. J. D. Thompson, "Organizations and Output Transactions," *American Journal of Sociology,* LXVIII (November, 1962), p. 320.

[37] This development suggests more of an "emergent process" than a cause-effect or mutual interaction course. Although causal relationships can be demonstrated between location use and feedback as well as affective processes, the overall evolution was one of a complex unified supportive system. Cf. Buckley, *Sociology and Modern Systems Theory,* pp. 80ff.

CHAPTER IV

THE DIABETIC CLINIC: A FAMILY BASED IMPROVISING ORGANIZATION

The identity of the diabetes clinic as supportive component in a coping system was underscored by the fact that a number of families utilizing the services were active members of local diabetic associations. The fathers of these families were frequently present at clinic sessions, [1] and these families were quite successful in gaining the attention and time of hospital personnel. Family involvement in the associations suggested their commitment to coping with the life-cycle issue posed by the child's illness.[2]

The clinic's orientation was influenced by its small size, by the nature of the illness, and by the treatment procedures adopted by the hospital. It had a rather intimate and family-oriented atmosphere. It was attended by only about fifteen families during a four-hour session on one afternoon of each week. Many of the families had been coming over a period of years and were well known to the members of the clinic staff; personal relationships among the families themselves were also evident.

[1] The frequent attendance of fathers of families active in voluntary health associations was also noted in the arthritis and cystic fibrosis clinics.

[2] Cf. M. Voysey, "Offiicial Agents and the Legitimation of Suffering," *Sociological Review,* NS XX (November, 1972), pp. 533-551. For a discussion of the identity problems of families dealing with chronic children's disabilities, and the resources employed in coping with these problems.

However, the part-time status of the clinic severely hampered its effectiveness. This was reflected in complaints of families about their unsuccessful attempts to reach physicians and nurses outside of clinic hours. The staff attempted to overcome the serious organizational problems of the clinic by adopting a warm interpersonal style. But despite good rapport between staff and families, there was evidence of failure in the delivery of health services.

IV-1. The Dominance of the Waiting Room[3]

The physical make-up of the clinic, which occupied one floor of a drab century-old building, contributed a unique atmosphere to the setting.[4] The entry was dominated by a waiting room about twenty-five feet in width and about thirty-five in length. Along three sides of the reception area were simple wooden benches with a few scattered tables on which magazines for children and parents were available. Off to the right as one entered the reception area a short corridor led to two examination rooms, an office used by the dietician, a laboratory and a washroom. At the entrance to the corridor and to one side was a small alcove containing the clerk's desk.[5]

About three-quarters of the total area was public in character. From the entrance to the waiting room, the administration desk and corridor were readily visible and were not available for private purposes.

[3] An earlier analysis of location of interaction in the diabetic and orthopedic clinics is presented in F. D. Powell, "A Concept of Structurated and Destructurated Group Roles: An Initial Empirical Reduction," *Social Science and Medicine,* IV (September, 1970), pp. 321-327.

[4] Literature pertaining to the ecology of organizations includes: E. Goffman, *The Presentation of Self in Everyday Life.* New York: Doubleday, 1959; E. Goffman, *Asylums: Essays on the Social Situation of Mental Patients and Other Inmates,* Chicago: Aldine, 1970; E. Goffman, *Behavior in Public Places; Notes on the Social Organization of Gatherings,* New York: Free Press Paperback, 1968; A. Hawley, *Human Ecology: A Theory of Community Structure,* New York: Ronald Press, 1950; S. M. Lyman and M. B. Scott, "Territoriality: A Neglected Sociological Dimension," *A Sociology of the Absurd,* New York: Appleton-Century-Crofts, 1970; F. Terrien and D. Mills, "The Effect of Changing Size Upon the Structure of Organizations," *American Sociological Review,* XX (February, 1955), pp. 11-13; O. D. Duncan and T. F. Schnore, "Cultural Behavioral and Ecological Perspectives in the Study of Social Organization," *American Journal of Sociology,* LXV (September, 1959), pp. 132-146; R. Sommer, "Studies in Personal Space," *Sociometry,* XXII (September, 1959), pp. 247-260; W. R. Rosengren and S. De Vault, "The Sociology of Time and Space in an Obstetrical Ward" in Eliot Freidson, ed., *The Hospital in Modern Society,* New York: The Free Press, 1963, pp. 266-291.

[5] *See Figure B-III-1, p. 34.*

The dominance of public or front areas[6] was closely connected with the organizational functioning of the clinic. The medical director was not as senior in point of hospital service as were the physicians in charge of the surgical and cystic fibrosis clinics. Additional staff consisted of three residents, a head nurse, a dietician and a clerk.

The small number of families at clinic sessions, the limited size of the staff, and the physical make-up of the clinic contributed to an informal atmosphere. This informality was highlighted by the practice of staff members, including physicians, of carrying on some of their activities with families in the waiting room. For example, physicians would frequently come into the waiting room to consult the clinic clerk on upcoming family appointments. While these arrangements were being made conversations between physicians and family members would commonly take place. These contacts between families and doctors were frequently of a social character. Sometimes, however, the medical staff used this location for inquiries about the progress of the child since the last clinic visit. These informal chats before going to the examination rooms produced a relaxed feeling on the part of family members. At the end of interviews doctors would sometimes accompany families back into the waiting room and spend some time talking with them before they left the clinic.[7]

If a special contact occurred with the clinic dietician, a similar procedure was followed. She would greet the family in the waiting room, and talk briefly there, before inviting them into her office to go over the details of the child's diet. These meetings would also often conclude with some final discussion in the waiting room.

The result was that for much of the time during clinic sessions there were several members of the staff engaged in conversation with different families in the reception area, in the corridor, or at the administration desk. The presence of the clerk, with whom appointments with physicians for subsequent visits were arranged, also helped establish the waiting room as a focal point of interaction between staff and family members.[8]

[6] Cf. Goffman, *The Presentation of Self in Everyday Life*. Cf. also Rosengren and De Vault, *op. cit.*, for discussion of use of "front" areas and "back" areas in an obstetrical ward. Cf. also parallel work of R. Pill, "Space and Social Structure in Two Children's Wards," *Sociological Review* XV NS(July, 1967), pp. 179-192.

[7] An exact count was not made of these appearances by physicians in the waiting room, but the recurrence of this behavior was frequently commented on by the observers and other members of the research team.

[8] The ecological structure of these waiting room groups conforms to Sommer's definition of "personal space" in which there are no marked, stationary limits, but in which the human body is the center, and space moves with the

The dominance of the reception room as a care center[9] for activities between staff and families was particularly marked in the case of the nurse. Of all nursing contact with families, 57% was carried on in the waiting room area. This location was used for carrying on health teaching of families and in particular for the instruction of children in the autonomous handling of the illness.[10]

The waiting room was an appropriate place for health teaching activities. The presence of several members of the staff had a legitimizing effect and established this as an appropriate location for health services. In particular the presence of physicians in the area gave validity to the waiting room as a fitting place for health team duties.[11] This support by physicians and other staff made possible a relaxed and informal tone with children and families. Thus there was greater tendency to focus on home-related issues in public than in private medical areas.[12]

The waiting room was also appropriate to the autonomy theme of diabetic health teaching. Since family members tended to predominate there and the furnishings, though simple, were for their convenience it seemed a natural place in which to emphasize the autonomous management of the illness.[13]

persons involved. This mobile, personal factor was related to the issue of autonomy which was stressed in health teaching. Cf. Sommer, "Studies in Personal Space," *Sociometry,* XXII (September, 1959), pp. 247-260.

[9] The proliferation of student centers on university campuses suggests a parallel need for locationally differentiated forums of care in the educational context.

[10] Cf. Appendix B, Table Ib, for figures on percentages in the first year in the other clinics, showing that only the cystic fibrosis clinic with 87% exceeded diabetic in waiting room contact.

[11] This informal character is consistent with Goffman's designation of the team as arising from interaction rather than from external structural demands. Cf. E. Goffman, *The Presentation of Self in Everyday Life,* p. 104.

[12] Cf. Table Ib in Appendix B, showing that 11% of home and life scope problems occurred in the waiting room and corridor while only 2% of such home-rlated activities took place in examination rooms.

[13] According to Goffman "decoration and permanent fixtures in a place" where a "particular performance" is found may tend "to fix a kind of spell over it." This "spell" of the waiting room furnishings, plus the constant presence of families there as the major grouping, produced an informal atmosphere favorable to the "performance" of autonomy teaching. Cf. E. Goffman, *The Presentation of Self in Everyday Life,* Edinburgh: University of Edinburgh, Social Science Research Center, monograph No. 2, 1956, p. 124. The atmosphere of social support found in the waiting room appears similar to that of the obstetrical admitting room as described in Rosengren and De Vault, "The Sociology of Time and Space in an Obstetrical Ward" in Freidson, ed., *The Hospital in Modern Society,* p. 274.

For both children and parents, the presence of other families had a supportive influence. More than in the examination room, families appeared to be at ease in a setting where they could feel that their problems were similar to those of other families whom they had grown to know through previous visits. As a result of the social support provided by the waiting room situation family members and staff felt less isolated in their efforts to deal with the problems of the illness.

The reception area though a public place was also a location for personal contact. During the normal progress of a clinic session, about fifteen persons were usually engaged in conversation in the waiting room, at the administration desk and in the corridor areas. The occupants of this public area broke up into diverse groups of family members and staff. One conversation might involve a family arranging with the clinic clerk for a return visit. A second discussion would, perhaps, be going on between a physician and another family receiving instructions at the conclusion of a visit to the examination room. Another conference might be taking place at the same time between the dietician and a mother about preparation of meals and the need for a varied but not too rigid diabetic diet. Talk would also often be in process between members of several families awaiting an opportunity to see one of the staff.

This busy scene, with its relaxed and easy pace of activities, provided a favorable setting for health teaching by the nurse. It was a common area available for the discussion of the specialized needs of individual families. The setting provided an atmosphere of social support for family members and staff engaged in discussing specific details of the diabetic regimen. A sense of social solidarity pervaded the public areas adjacent to the waiting room. This social solidarity provided support to the nurse and to families. The feeling was communicated that the problems being discussed were not totally unique to each family. At the same time conversations going on in other groups in the waiting room and at the administration desk permitted a sufficient degree of privacy for contacts between staff and families.

A structure of permeable boundaries existed between the various groups in the reception areas and corridor. The existence of these permeable boundaries permitted a considerable degree of freedom of expression and intimacy in the interaction.[14]

[14] Permeable boundaries between the various interactions relate to Goffman's analysis of "accessible engagements" or "free engagements carried on in the presence of outsiders." The requirement of "civil inattention" appears not to have prevailed, however, in the diabetic waiting room. The similarity of problems of the various families and a relatively low level of anxiety permitted a casual amount of general awareness on the part of outsiders. This general casual awareness contributed to the support structure without involv-

The informal contact that occurred in the waiting room between staff members also gave rise to specific forms of collaboration and chance alliances between the nurse, physicians and administrative staff of the hospital.[15] Collaboration was exemplified by plans made between the nurse and the clinic chief for joint efforts in assisting specific families. Support for the nurse's activities in the waiting room was exhibited by questions of health teaching procedures directed to her by younger physicians. In some instances, where families had particularly complex problems, the nurse was able to take the initiative in enlisting the assistance of physicians, administrative staff and nursing personnel from other clinics in mobilizing help. Her activities in the waiting room were greatly enhanced by the opportunity for frequent informal contact with members of the staff. The waiting room as a common area of health delivery perceptibly reduced status differences between physicians and other staff members.[16]

IV-2. Examination Room as an Area of Legitimation

Although most family contacts took place in the waiting room, a substantial portion of time was spent with families in the examination rooms. In fact, 35% of interaction took place in the examination rooms, often in the company of one of the staff physicians.[17]

These contacts with physicians played a role in legitimizing nursing activities. This was especially the case with family interviews involving the clinic chief. Family teaching by the nurse had the direct endorsement of the chief, and the nurse appeared to use these interviews to reinforce this approval. This was done by providing information on the progress of families and children in handling the illness. In a number of sequences the nurse and the chief functioned as an effective team instructing families on insulin management and on keeping accurate records.

ing direct intrusion into the conversation. Cf. E. Goffman, *Behavior in Public Places,* especially, "Communication Boundaries," pp. 151-165.

[15] The data from the diabetes clinic suggests that physicians can be protected from unnecessary harassment by families in the waiting room by a sensitive health team approach.

[16] This lowering of status barriers in the waiting room suggested the conditions of milieu therapy proposed by E. Goffman, *The Presentation of Self in Everyday Life,* p. 199. The characteristics of the waiting room as an area of social support for family and staff appear similar to those of the therapeutic milieu as specified by Rapoport. Cf. Robert N. Rapoport (with Rhona Rapoport and I. Rosow), *Community as Doctor: New Perspectives on a Therapeutic Community,* London. Tavistock Publications, 1960.

[17] Cf. Table Ib, Appendix B.

The examination room was also a place for individual contact between the nurse and physicians. These conferences were used to review family diabetic records and to plan the teaching procedures to be followed by the nurse. In these meetings the nurse was able to maintain a rather independent position in relation to physicians. Although at times the latter would not follow the nurse's suggestions for treating medical problems, the nurse maintained her autonomy with physicians by virtue of closer acquaintance with families.[18]

The legitimacy of the waiting room as an area for health activities was attenuated by the use of the examination rooms by physicians as the prime medical area. Although physicians did spend some time in the waiting room with families, the nurse appeared to acquire status through her contacts in the examination room with doctors, particularly with the chief of the clinic.[19]

IV-3. Part-Time Status of a Polycentered System

The need to legitimize nursing activities was symptomatic of the clinic's instability within the hospital structure. The clinic was restricted in its operations to one afternoon a week. Its personnel, including the nurse, spent only a small portion of their working time serving the needs of the families.[20] The consequence was that the diabetic service did not loom large in the political make-up of the hospital. This was so because the clinic was not closely affiliated with any of the more powerful hospital units, such as was the case with arthritis.

Moreover, the use of the waiting room for health related activities departed from standard practices employed in the high status services of the outpatient department. The surgical clinics followed uniform procedure in giving priority to the use of examination rooms for family contact with physicians and nurses.[21] It was also the practice of surgeons to avoid the waiting room areas whenever possible.

[18] The autonomy of diabetic nursing also was related to the issue of institutional discrepancy. Cf. below V-9.

[19] This need to acquire status by way of contact with physicians in the examination room emphasized the character of the waiting room as a marginal region devoted to care functions in the clinic. This regional character was based on its separation from the examination room by "barriers to perception." Cf. Goffman, *The Presentation of Self in Everyday Life,* p. 106.

[20] The nurse, herself diabetic, spent four days a week in the surgical services of the outpatient department.

[21] Comparative percentages of waiting room use for family contact as given in Table Ib in Appendix B were 57% in diabetic, 87% in cystic fibrosis, 6% in orthopedic and 2% in arthritis during the first year. These figures indicate the radical departure of diabetes and cystic fibrosis from the practices of the surgical clinics.

In consequence, the use of the waiting room by the diabetic nurse for family oriented activities violated usual patterns.[22] The appearance of physicians in the waiting room in diabetes also departed from institutional norms.[23] Although the presence of physicians and other clinic staff gave support to waiting room activities, this support did not constitute full institutional acceptance.[24] It was necessary also to maintain contact with physicians in the examination room to fully legitimize nursing activities in the waiting room.[25]

The diabetic clinic was thus a polycentered system, with the waiting room, devoted to the autonomy teaching of children, assuming primary significance ecologically as care center of the clinic. Unfortunately, the part-time status of the clinic, seriously limited the effectiveness of the support provided to families through autonomy teaching.

IV-4. Inquiry Teaching Approach

Family control of treatment was sought through an inquiry teaching method adopted by the nursing staff. This teaching approach was encouraged by the medical chief. Physician support was indicated by questions on teaching procedures directed to the nurse by the chief and by younger members of the medical staff.

The inquiry approach was evidenced by efforts of the staff to obtain answers from children on their understanding and management of the illness. Owing to the stress placed on the child's control of treatment, it was appropriate as a means of determining their capacity to manage. Questions were directed to children rather than to parents; children

[22] This avoidance was only overcome by the crowded and under-staffed conditions in the old orthopedic clinic which compelled physicians to become involved reluctantly in disputes with families in claims for limited services. Adjudication of these disputes tended to take place at the appointment desk.

[23] The diabetic and cystic fibrosis clinics represent a departure from a medical model of performance of cure and care functions in staff-defined area (e. g., the examination rooms) and as such were locationally complex systems. The orthopedic and arthritis clinics as staff-based health care services were locationally more simple systems. Cf. W. Buckley, *Sociology and Modern Systems Theory*, pp. 46-50.

[24] The need for such support networks in a polycentered system such as diabetes appears to conform to Buckley's requirements of information links in complex systems, and of interactive needs in respect to the environment in open systems.

[25] In terms of this index of examination room contact, nursing activities were the most legitimate in the arthritis clinic with 97% and in orthopedics with 83% family examination room contact; whereas diabetes was less legitimized with 35% of such contact, and cystic fibrosis least with 8%. Cf. Appendix B, Table Ib.

from the age of four were expected to have a grasp of treatment procedures.[26]

IV-5. Inquiry Methods and Anxiety: An Example of Family Dynamics

From an early age, depending on individual maturity and stability of the family structure, questions would be directed to the child. These pertained to keeping a diet book, understanding the effects on blood sugar of various types of food, managing insulin injections and reactions, and following a reasonable diabetic diet.

The inquiry procedure frequently brought to light emotional difficulties within the family as illustrated by a passage from interaction with an eight-year-old girl and her mother. The child was being questioned about her ability to manage insulin injections. She had already demonstrated her ability to understand the meaning of various colors used in carrying out urine tests. The nurse praised the child for being able to manage this task, and then began to question her about insulin injections.

Nurse to child: Do you give your own insulin? Do you draw it up?

Child to nurse: I'm scared. [Child laughs.]

Mother to nurse: She doesn't know how to draw it up. She knows how to give it. I have to draw it up.

Child to mother: I know how you do it, Mama.

Mother to child: You can't draw it up the right way.

Child to mother: Yes sir.

Mother to child: You told me you didn't know how to do it.

Child to mother: I told you that I could.

[26] This emphasis on patient understanding of the illness, personal approach by staff and unauthoritarian style of health teaching closely parallels the treatment of glaucoma as specified by Riffenburgh. Cf. R. S. Riffenburgh, "Doctor-patient Relationship in Glaucoma Therapy," *Archives of Ophthalmology,* LXXV (July, 1966), p. 204. From about four years the children attending the clinic were instructed in the effects of diet on the sugar content of the blood. Cf. Szasz and Hollander and also S. W. Bloom for discussion of variant models of approach to patient activity in dealing with illness. Cf. also E. Miller for discussion of "warehouse" vs. "horticultural" models of patient care, *Research Monograph,* The Tavistock Institute of Human Relations, London, 1972. Cf. S. W. Bloom, *The Doctor and His Patient; A Sociological Interpretation,* New York: Free Press, 1965. Cf. T. Szasz and M. Hollander, "A Contribution to the Philosophy of Medicine," *A.M.A. Archives of Internal Medicine,* Vol. 97, No. 5, (May, 1956), p. 585.

Nurse *(speaking to child while mother says something inaudible in the background to the child)* What if I bring in a syringe and a bottle . . . whether you can or not? It's not . . .

Child to nurse: I've practiced with an orange before at camp.

Nurse to child: Did you go to Clara Barton camp?

[The mother interjected a comment concerning the fact that . . . she was surprised that the child could draw up the insulin. This was followed by a brief discussion of the child's plans to return to a summer camp for diabetic children.]

Mother to nurse: She gave it to herself.

Nurse to child: Did you give it to yourself at camp? Where did you give it? In your leg? You should try to give it at home when you come back from camp. Next time . . .

Child *(interrupting nurse):* Yeh, but I get scared. Because I didn't do it for a long time!

Nurse to child: So when you go to camp, they will have you doing it and when you come home it's going to be a lot easier for you to keep on doing it. What if you wanted to go over to a girl friend's at night? Who's going to give it to you the next morning? Pretty soon you're going to start wanting to do these things and you can't drag your mother along every place you go. Right? If you can give it to an orange you can give it to yourself. You don't mind when your mother gives it, right? It's not that you're afraid of the needle?

Child to nurse: It hurts when my mother gives it to me. It doesn't hurt when my daddy gives it to me. [Child laughs.]

Mother to nurse: That's all I hear laterly, when you give it it hurts and when dad gives it it doesn't.

Nurse to child: Where does your father give it?

Child to nurse: In my bum.

Nurse to child: Where does your mother give it?

Child to nurse: In my bum. [Child laughs.]

Nurse to child: What about your leg? What about your tummy?

IV-6. Emphasis on Medical Scope

In the interaction of the nurse with this mother and young girl several different types of problems were involved. First, there were the technical problems of injections, and of rotation of sites to achieve desired effects from the insulin. At a different level, there were dynamics within the family in its attempts to cope with the problems of the illness. These problems included the child's fears of the injections. These fears were controlled in the camp situation and when injections were given by the father, but recurred in the home situation when the child tried to give them herself or received them from the mother. A third kind of issue was posed when the nurse raised the question of what might happen if the child wanted to "go over to a girl friend's at night?" Here the nurse raised implications of the illness in life-cycle terms and tried to persuade the child that eventually she would have to manage the illness without the help of her parents.

Through the interaction that took place with this family a pattern to the scope of the issues can be discerned. The first issue, the knowledge of how to conduct urine testing, was technical in nature. Discussions of such matters as effects on blood sugar content of carbohydrates and sweets were similarly technical. The child's responses indicated that she was able to understand most of these matters.

The nurse then moved the discussion to the subject of injections. In the course of this questioning a conflict emerged between the child and the mother, from which the nurse attempted to escape by returning the discussion to a technical level. Later on, when the life cycle issue of independence from parents was raised, and fear of the "needle" was expressed, a new conflict was uncovered involving the child's preference for receiving injections from her father rather than from her mother.[27] Here again the nurse attempted to avoid an area of family conflict about injections, by shifting the discussion to the rotation of injection sites. As the nurse brought up specific technical areas the social and emotional problems of the family tended to surface. The nurse shifted the focus of discussion to a new technical area when these emotional problems arose.[28]

[27] The unwillingness of the nurse to become involved in family dynamics suggests Brodey and Hayden's comment that staff members may often be impeded in dealing with such problems by intra-staff difficulties. Thus in the second year, when diabetes nursing was more free in relation to physicians, family problems, including fathers' roles within families were more directly handled. Cf. W. M. Brodey and M. Hayden, "Intrateam Reactions: Their Relations to the Conflicts of the Family in Treatment," *American Journal of Orthopsychiatry,* XXVII (April, 1957), pp. 349-355.

[28] The dynamics of this family in relating to the nurse is reminiscent of Piaget's comment that "cooperation is at first the source of criticism and individualism." The nurse in attempting to obtain the "cooperation" of the child evoked "criticism" of the mother for her unwillingness to provide support in performing the diabetic tasks. The preference for the father's assistance

IV-7. Autonomy Theme and Conflict with Family Social Patterns

The expectation of the hospital that children should become autonomous in managing the illness ran counter to patterns existing in many families. Family resistance to this idea is exemplified by a discussion with two young boys of five and eight years, who came to the clinic with their mother. The nurse in this interview was trying to persuade one of the boys to teach his younger brother how to test urine.

Nurse to older brother: But you help him. You teach him . . . You teach him how to play cowboys, don't you? And you teach him how to do things you want to do.

Older brother to nurse: I never play with him.

Nurse to older brother: You never play with your own brother?

Older brother to nurse: No. I have Billy Jones, and me and him both have stingrays, and we ride them around.

Nurse to older brother: But you never play with Charles? Not even at night?

Older brother to nurse: No.

Nurse to older brother: When you're in the house? I don't believe that.

Older brother to nurse: Sometimes I play with him, and sometimes I don't.

Nurse to older brother: Okay. And you teach him, you teach him your games, so teach him this one.

Older brother to nurse: I can't teach him how to ride a bike.

Nurse to older brother: No, but you can teach him how to test his urine. You can teach him how to pick up five drops of urine and five drops of water.

Older brother to nurse: No, ten drops.

Nurse to older brother: Ten drops of water. You're right! [Everybody laughs.] You're smarter than you think you are. Will you try?

Nurse to younger brother: What about you, Charles, are you going to let him teach you?

suggests the "individualism" which Piaget associates with "moral development." Cf. Jean Piaget, "Social Factors in Moral Development", in Harold Proshansky and Bernard Seidenberg, eds., *Basic Studies in Social Psychology*, New York: Holt, Rinehart and Winston, 1965 (Reprinted from J. Piaget, *The Moral Judgement of the Child*, New York: The Free Press of Glencoe, 1932), p. 281.

Charles: [Giggles.]

Mother to nurse: He's tried it a few times but he messes up on it.

Nurse to mother: On the drops?

Mother to nurse: It's easier doing it myself. [Laughs.]

Nurse to mother: Have him do it a couple of times . . . I . . . you know, it probably would be easier but it is best that he start doing some things before he gets into school.

This passage indicates the resistance put up by this family to efforts of the nurse to foster the younger child's autonomy. When an effort was made to negotiate a tentative agreement between the two brothers to work on the injections, the mother resisted the arrangement. The attempt to persuade the mother to see that the child mastered the task before he entered school seemed inconclusive.

This interaction shows a conflict between the goals of the hospital and the attitude of the family in the management of the illness by the child. From the perspective of the staff the children's management of the illness was a clear and reasonable goal. The staff saw the child growing up and recognized his need to become independent of the parents. There was also a tendency to equate a rational understanding with the ability to assume responsibility in carrying out the task. When the older child showed inadvertently that he knew how to perform the urine test the nurse assumed that he was "smart" enough to teach the urine test procedures to his brother. With the mother the nurse assumed the rational point of view in stating the need for the child to be able to do urine testing before his entry into school.

However, the mother's response that it was "easier doing it myself" expressed a different attitude toward the issue of autonomy. This mother, like a number of the families visiting the diabetic clinic, had several children suffering from the illness. The activities associated with the management of diabetes, along with the arrangement of periodic visits to the clinic, were a heavy demand upon the attention and time of these families. In such circumstances there was a strong tendency for the mother to retain responsibility for the management of the diabetic routines. In the face of pressure from the staff to establish the child's responsibility for the care of the condition, there was resistance and maintenance of dependency patterns due to time constraints. In practical terms, what was "best" for the child, yielded to what was "easier" for the family.

IV-8. Improvising Trends in the Diabetic Clinic

As a health delivery system that operated a separate care center in the waiting room area of the clinic, the diabetic services may be classified strategically and locationally as a family-based coping sub-system. In terms of its interactive or tactical patterns the diabetic clinic displayed some features of an improvising system.

Improvisational patterns include a tendency toward heightened emotional tone, a moderate degree of structuring of interactive roles, a tendency to discuss non-technical or home-related issues, and an emphasis on family initiative. The interaction in the diabetic clinic displayed some of these improvising elements, while other features were more ritualized in nature.

IV-9. Diffused Affect and Autonomy Teaching

An analysis has been made of affective behavior linking it conceptually with goal-oriented activities in the clinics. This analysis (as instanced by the emergence of affective channelling in arthritis) was useful in analyzing the clinics as improvising interactive systems. In the case of diabetes, staff emphasis was on the attempt to elicit from children a willingness to undertake autonomous management of the disease. In line with this approach there was a close connection (as revealed by cross-tabulation of the data) between small talk and courtship on the one hand, and between courtship and both feedback opportunity and service on the other. Thus strong interrelationships were recorded for the conjunction of small talk and courtship at high intensity; while similarly strong relationships were shown between intense levels of courtship and high intensities of feedback opportunity and service.[29]

The affective pattern in the clinic suggested one of affective diffusion. That is, when work was being done, lavish amounts of emotional expression were employed. On the other hand, when work activities were not in progress, a sharply lesser abundance of feelings was in evidence. Although the absolute level of affect during non-work sequences was comparable to that in other clinics (e.g., cystic fibrosis[30])

[29] Cf. Appendix B, Table VIII, Col. 5, showing strong concurrence of high intensities of small talk and courtship (expression ratio = 4.394); courtship and opportunity for feedback (expression ratio = 3.691); and courtship and service (expression ratio = 2.774). Thus a sharp predominance of high over low emotional expression prevailed while task activities were in progress (yielding an overall expression ratio of 3.620. Cf. Appendix B, Table VII, Col. 4). This contrasted rather sharply with intense feelings expressed during non-work related situations. Thus comparatively low levels of affect tended to emerge during socially defined sequences (as indicated by a *relatively* low reservoir ratio of 0.823; Cf. Appendix B, Table VII, Col. 3).

[30] Cf. Appendix B, Table VII, Col. 3.

GRAPH G-IV-9

Components of Affective Behavior in the Diabetes and Orthopedic Clinics during the First Year

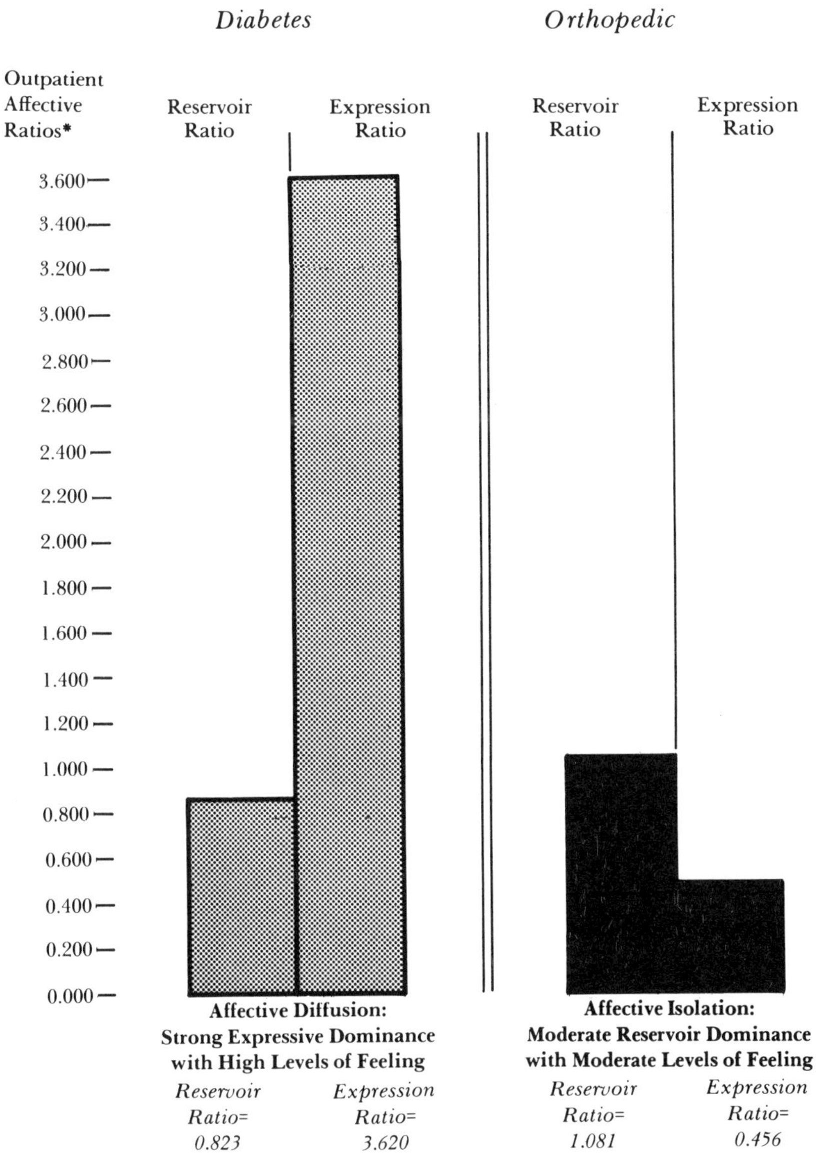

**Based on ratios presented in Table VII, Appendix B, p. 207.*

the reduction of feeling between work oriented and socially defined situations was the greatest observed in the course of the research.[31]

Viewing emotional levels during non-work activities as a social reservoir a great discrepancy occurred between this level and that displayed during task performance.[32] The fact that feelings were intensively engaged during goal-oriented sequences, indicated the important role played by emotional expression during the autonomy teaching interviews. The *relatively* low level of feelings shown outside of work situations suggested that emotions were intensified during the work sequences, with comparatively reduced reserves maintained for casual contact.

The sharp differences in the amounts of feelings employed during work and non-work sequences may be seen in Graph G-IV-9. The pattern of affective diffusion that marked diabetes interaction was in contrast with that in the orthopedic clinic. As shown in the graph, orthopedic interaction was characterized by a rise of feelings during periods of rest, with restricted emotions during work activities. This latter pattern of affective isolation was strikingly different from that of the diabetic clinic.

IV-10. Discordant Interactive Elements

Certain features of the interactive network displayed ritual rather than improvising tendencies. Among these were the dominance of medical scope and of staff initiative. These trends were derived from the precise medical technology available in diabetes, and from the efforts of the staff to inculcate an understanding of this technology. Thus overall 87% of all interaction with families took place at medical scope. Moreover, staff initiation amounted to 71.5%, with families accounting for only 28.5% of the initiative.

However, in the waiting room families initiated 49.3% of the home scope interaction, whereas in the examination room family home scope initiative declined to 24.4%. The effect of the waiting room as care center of the clinic was to deritualize the interactive network. More

[31] As evidenced by a difference of opinion and reservoir ratios of 2.797. Ibid, Col. 5.

[32] This pattern of affective diffusion suggests a different approach to the analysis of feeling from that of the intimacy scale developed by Samuel and Mannheim insofar as "intimacy" appears to describe emotions expressed apart from task activities. According to the present approach intense "intimacy" would tend to coincide with "isolated affect." Cf. Y. Samuel and B. H. Mannheim, "A Multidimensional Approach toward a Typology of Bureaucracy," *Administrative Science Quarterly,* XV (March, 1970), pp. 216-228.

GRAPH-H-IV-10

Role Structuring in the Diabetes and Orthopedic Clinics during the First Year
(medical scope interaction*)

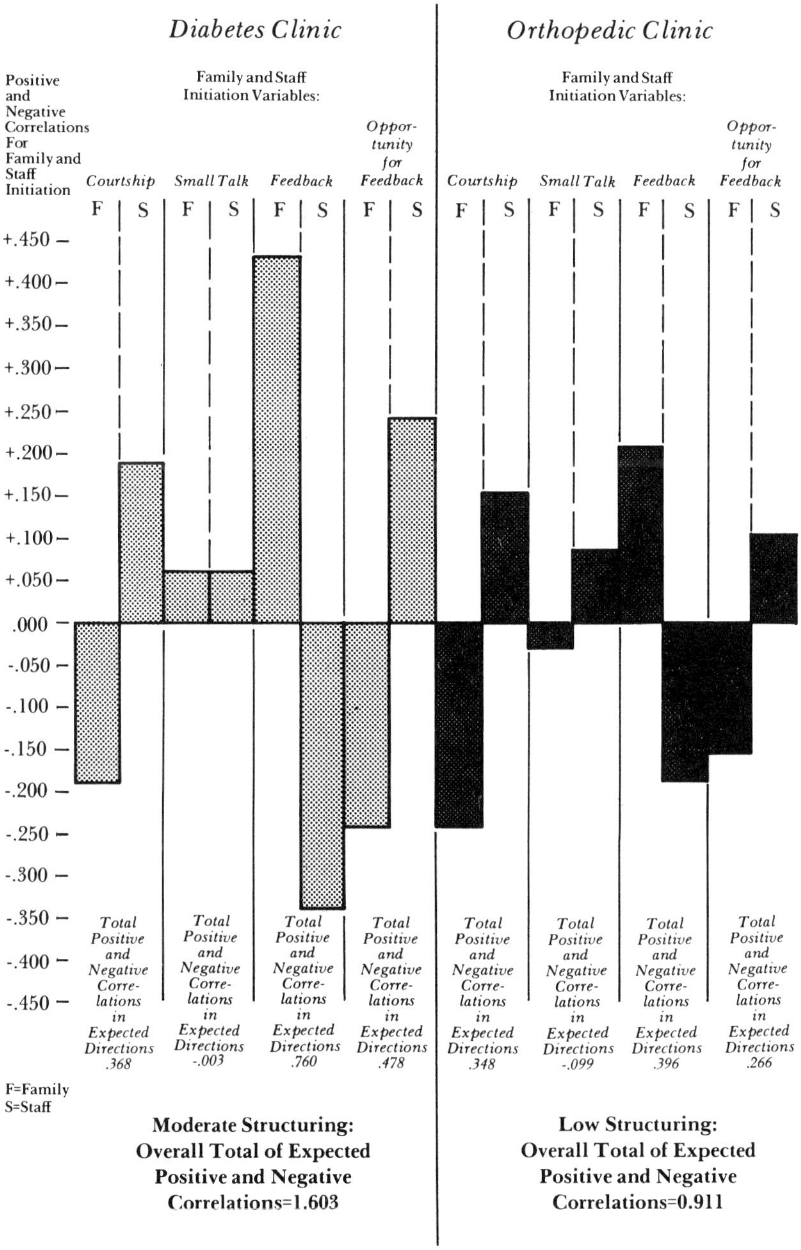

**Based on lagged correlations as presented in Appendix B, Tables IV and V, pp. 205-6.*

home scope problems and more family initiative were manifest there. The atmosphere of the waiting room with its informal relationships between staff and families contributed toward improvising tendencies in the interactive pattern of the clinic. The strong affective and inquiry patterns in the public areas moderated staff dominated technical ritual elements.[33]

An analysis of feedback-related activities also indicated a rather clearly structured interactive system.[34] The didactic approach adopted in diabetes resulted in a clear demarcation of interactive types. Staff in an autonomy teaching capacity were active in initiating courtship and feedback opportunity. Families in responding to this didactic procedure initiated small talk and offered feedback to the staff.

The fixed patterning of roles is evident from Graph H-IV-10. A sharp contrast may be seen with the orthopedic clinic where no such structuring of activities around autonomy teaching prevailed. The marked reduction in staff-family differences in feedback and opportunity for feedback, suggested greater reciprocity in communication in orthopedics than in diabetes.

IV-11. Discrepant Improvisation and Weak Responsiveness

The diabetic clinic as an interactive network combined both improvising and ritual elements. High levels of affective diffusion were combined with a well defined interactive differentiation and an emphasis on staff initiated medical scope problems. This inconsistency in interactive components was associated with a low level of responsiveness as measured by sensitivity during feedback processes.[35]

The unresponsive feedback processes are highlighted by a comparison with the orthopedic clinic as shown in Graph J-IV-11. In the latter

[33] Cf. Appendix B, Table II. The strong trends toward home-related discussion in the waiting room are consonant with the milieu effects, pointed out by Sussman, on outpatient satisfaction. Cf. M. B. Sussman *et al.*, *The Walking Patient,* p. 73.

[34] Thus by use of a correlation analysis staff-assigned interactive roles of courtship and opportunity for feedback were compared with family-related roles of small talk and providing of feedback. Combined differences of staff from family initiation in the first two activities, and family from staff initiation in the latter types of interaction were the largest found in any of the clinics (a combined difference in correlations of 1.603 in medical scope interaction). Cf. Appendix B, Tables IV & V, for comparison with other clinics.

[35] Thus, staff response to prior feedback opportunity was only 18.5%, while family sensitivity of response to prior inquiries amounted to only 13.8%; the unweighted average feedback responsiveness of 16.2% was the lowest recorded in any of the outpatient services. Cf. Appendix B, Table VI.

clinic both families and staff showed a greater willingness to respond during feedback exchanges. The reduced structuring of roles in orthopedics, as compared with diabetes during the first year, was a factor contributing to the effectiveness of the orthopedic feedback procedures.

The weak diabetic feedback pattern was traceable to the extreme medical and technical emphasis adopted in the teaching sequences, along with staff dominance of interaction. Families had little opportunity to introduce home problems and thus to initiate a reciprocal process that would result in greater sensitivity during feedback ex-

GRAPH J-IV-11

Feedback Responsiveness* by Families and Staff in the Diabetes and Orthopedic Clinics during the First Year

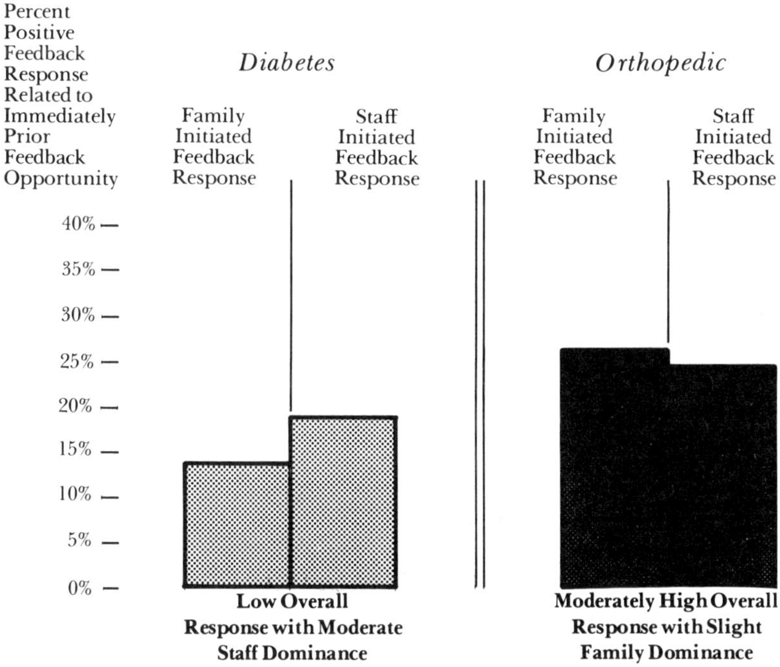

Diabetes	Orthopedic
Average (unweighted) Family-Staff Feedback Response= 16.2%	*Average (unweighted) Family-Staff Feedback Response=25.2%*
Specific Feedback Response	*Specific Feedback Response*
Family=13.8%	*Family=26.2%*
Staff=18.5%	*Staff=24.2%*

**Based on lagged regression analysis of data presented in Table VI, Appendix B, p. 207.*

change. Staff members came programmed, as it were, to engage in health teaching of diabetic routine. The efforts of families to inject home-related problems were brushed aside as irritants impeding the teaching process. The effect of the informality of the waiting room was to reduce somewhat the ritualized patterns of a tight medical technology. This informality, however, was not sufficient to initiate a sensitive feedback process. The diabetic service in the old clinic building was a family-based coping sub-system displaying ritualized features of discordant and non-responsive improvising social interaction.

The part-time status of the diabetic service did not provide an adequate organizational basis for the support of families through direct autonomy teaching of children in the clinic. In fact the effort to establish a program of autonomy teaching in the clinic represented an underutilization of community health resources available to families. The initiative that was undertaken in the new clinic to involve community health teams was a more creative expression of support.

CHAPTER V

THE DIABETIC CLINIC: CHANGE IN A FAMILY BASED IMPROVISING ORGANIZATION

V-1. Physical and Organizational Changes

Seven months prior to the second period of observation the clinics of the outpatient department moved to a modern high rise building which had been constructed as an addition to the hospital facilities. The physical changes in the diabetic clinic were dramatic.

In place of the small, crowded waiting room with old wooden benches and a few tables, a large, modern reception area with comfortable and tastefully arranged couches and chairs had been installed. Modern carpeting and soundproof ceilings greatly reduced noise. Attractive play areas had been provided with tables, chairs and black boards. (See Figure C-III-1, page 34, above.)

Facing the waiting room, at the entrance to the medical areas of the clinic, was a large administration desk. In the administrative area, files and computerized information were available containing the medical history of families visiting the clinic. Leading from the waiting room on each side of the administration desk were two wide parallel corridors giving access to the medical areas of the clinic. Halfway down the corridors, a connecting hallway permitted easy flow of traffic through the medical sectors. Located along the outside edge of the building were examination rooms, physicians' offices and a nursing station. The interior portion of the medical area between the two corridors was devoted to a residents' room, laboratories and a dietician's office.

Organizational changes included the addition of a second clinic clerk to assist at the administration desk. The expanded clerical staff assumed new responsibilities, formerly carried out by nurses, in routing patients and their families through the clinic and in arranging for appointments. An additional part-time nursing assistant was introduced to help in technical matters and in providing aid to physicians.

Changes also took place among physicians attached to staff of the clinic. Principal among these was the decision of the chief of the clinic to leave the staff of the hospital a short time after the second period of formal observations. The medical director's decision had become known in the clinic and may have affected adversely the functioning of staff members. The complement of physicians serving the clinic was not increased, and actually declined relative to the new surgical services of the outpatient department.

V-2. Changes in Area Usage

In status and in size the diabetic clinic declined further in power and importance relative to some other outpatient services. No significant additional funds were allocated to the new clinic. Residents and interns serving in the hospital thought of diabetes as a garden variety illness. The teaching staff of the hospital did not regard diabetes as a primary area for medical learning and interns were not inclined to seek out the clinic as an area of interesting research or of career opportunities.

Moreover, physical and organizational trends in the diabetic department moved in a direction that was contrary to the type of health service approach that had been previously taken. Physically, this was expressed by the isolation of the waiting room from the medical areas of the clinic. A twenty-foot-long administration counter faced the waiting room where the clerical staff received families. Rear doors for staff led from the administrative area into the corridors and medical sectors. This arrangement facilitated the formal separation of the staff, especially physicians, from families awaiting services in the reception area.

This physical isolation was organizationally expressed by the failure of physicians to appear in the waiting room as a routine part of their services in the clinic.

In the new situation the absence of the physicians from the waiting room resulted in the isolation of the nursing staff in carrying out health teaching activities. To a large extent nurses continued to use the waiting room as the primary location for contact with families. There was evidence, however, that both clerical staff and physicians failed to accord to waiting room activities the status that had been given in the old clinic. A decline in the informality and warmth of the reception area was suggested by the new use of a public address system for calling families to the administration desk for appointments.

V-3. Community Orientation in the Diabetic Clinic

The isolation of the waiting room from some members of the staff was accompanied by a rise in nursing administrative activity in the interstitial areas of the clinic. These administrative involvements focused on contacts with health personnel inside and outside the hospital.

A widening range of health service contacts resulted from a community oriented effort by the diabetic nursing staff. The new policy involved the establishment of working relationships with visiting nurses' associations and school health departments in the communities where diabetic families resided. It also involved close working arrangements with hospital personnel including physicians and social workers. Plans for family assistance and guidance were adopted which involved collaboration between the hospital and community health services. Similar arrangements were worked out with members of school health departments for the needs of families. Assistance from physicians was sought for this community oriented policy. Despite severe problems the support of doctors was obtained in implementing this new socially oriented program.

V-4. Example of Community-Oriented Health Care

An example of the new community approach adopted toward families in the diabetic clinic is suggested by an interview that took place with a mother and her three-year-old son, along with three other young children, of whom only one was of school age. It is of interest that during the course of the interview a physician entered the room and, after about five minutes, left without having interrupted the discussion. After the conference, the physician was involved in planning the follow-up by a hospital social worker who had been assisting the family. The conversation, focused largely on the disciplining of the child, began with the nurse inquiring about the issue of "mothering":

Nurse to mother: How much mothering does he get? You know, how much time—I mean sure, with four children that you don't have enough time . . .

Mother to nurse *(interrupting her):* I give him a lot of love.

Nurse to mother: Can you spend, can you spend a half hour or some amount of time with when you just . . .

Mother to nurse *(interrupting again):* Yea, when I'm with him alone. He's very good. Don't touch that, Bart! [Now shouting at patient.] Bart!

Patient to mother: I'm sorry.

Mother to child: Don't do it!

Mother to nurse: You know, if I have to go someplace I leave the other kids, I only take him. He's good, you know. There are a lot of kids in the neighborhood that get too much attention, I mean . . . [Her comments are rendered inaudible by the children's noise.]

Mother to patient: Put that down!

Nurse to patient: That's a tape measure to see how big you are.

Patient to nurse: Big fat?

Nurse to patient: Hm hm.

Patient to nurse: I'm fat.

Nurse to patient: Let's see how big you are around the tummy. Show me.

Patient to nurse: No.

Nurse to mother: Look, it may be that he really wants some attention. And if you could or perhaps plan some projects for him to do around the house . . .

Mother to nurse: Well, look, he's got more toys, everything's around . . .

Nurse to mother *(interrupting her):* This, this, I don't know if this is what he's after, you know, the fact that of . . .

Mother to nurse: No, he just acts like this, he just does this like if I just go out of the house, he gets all upset. If we're out in the yard, I have to hold his hand.

Nurse to patient: That's a test tube, and would you please put it back for me.

Patient to nurse: Do you use these?

Nurse to patient: Please put it back. [Apparently starting to lose her patience.] Thank you very much.

[Observer's comment: A physician entered, sat listening for a few minutes, then left without any comment at 2:45. This three year old is a behavior and disciplinary problem to the mother. The nurse focused on this rather than on the diabetes because it seemed to be where the mother needed assistance. The nurse related to the child very effectively and I was hoping the mother would be perceptive enough to make this observation, but I don't think she did.[1] The nurse tried to impress the mother with the need for a consistency in following through on what she said. This she did. If she told the child not to do something or he would get a spanking, she followed through with spanking the child. The child showed symptoms of tension by periodically tightening up his lower jaw that would be consistent with his teeth grinding that the mother mentioned. The nurse referred the mother to the social worker because the children were sleeping with her and the husband in the children's bed.[2]]

Following this interview a conference took place in the clinic nursing office between the staff nurse, her assistant and the physician who had appeared earlier. It was agreed that the social worker who had been following this family should be contacted. The head nurse put through a call to the social worker, and described the problems of the family, including the disciplinary and sleeping arrangements. The physician actively cooperated in arranging for the social worker to contact the family before it ended the clinic visit.[3]

V-5. Community Orientation and Home Scope Issues

The focus of the attention was a series of home problems, rather than

[1] The observer's comment as to the difficulty of the nurse in conveying to the mother the need to "relate" more "effectively" to the child is associated with social class differences in regard to disciplinary matters as proposed by Kohn. Middle class parents emphasize obedience to internalized norms of control, whereas this mother seemed to rely upon external authority appeals. Cf. M. L. Kohn, *Class and Conformitory: A Study in Values,* Homewood, Illinois: Dorsey Press, 1969.

[2] The efforts of the nurse to assist the mother in relating more meaningfully to the child appear to have failed, though some progress may have been made in achieving greater consistency in disciplinary matters. This mixed pattern illustrates Thompson's observation on "heuristic-optional" interactions in which "the distinction between a process leading toward side transactions often is difficult to distinguish from one leading to transaction." Cf. J. D. Thompson, "Organizations and Output Transactions," *American Journal of Sociology,* LXVIII (November, 1962), p. 321.

[3] The facilitating action of the physician, along with his observation of a portion of the nurse's interaction with this family illustrates Thompson's comments on the supervisory role in relation to boundary-spanning personnel. The physician in arranging contact with social service for this family, at the request of the nurse, demonstrated "reinforcement of an output role" by "balancing rapport and treatment". Cf. J. D. Thompson, "Organizations and Output Transactions," *American Journal of Sociology,* LXVIII (November, 1962).

diabetes as a disease entity. In the judgment of the nurse, concurred in by the observer, it was the discipline and mothering of the child that bothered this parent, more than the technical handling of the illness. In addition there were serious problems of family disorganization that required the attention of the social work department. Although there had been efforts during the first year to involve the social services, they were made in terms of immediate crises. The sequence with this family indicated long range planning, as evidenced by the collaboration of the physician. By three-way teamwork between nurses, social workers and staff physicians, a comprehensive long-range care, focusing on home issues, was put in motion on behalf of this family.[4]

V-6. Diabetic Support

The comprehensive planning and sensitive approach adopted with this family suggested a new type of supportive effort in the clinic. In the first year a programmed approach limited to technical management had marked the teaching efforts in the clinic. In the second year as seen with this family and with a number of others, an effort was made to plan health services around the most pressing central family needs.

As reflected in interviews from the first year, failure to deal with family dynamics frequently resulted in ineffective efforts to convey technical diabetic instruction to children. In the case of this family, the observer noted the avoidance of diabetes as a "disease entity" and the nurse's focus on discipline and the broad array of human problems in the family. The approach involved the collaboration of a spectrum of personnel in the hospital and in the home community.

This health team approach focused on supportive help to the family. The assumption was made that without basic assistance in the underlying social organization of this family, technical management of the illness was impossible. Although the social problems were very complicated, equally difficult home situations had also been encountered in the first year. The fact that such problems were tackled in the new clinic signalled a new supportive approach. This effort to provide supportive assistance as a basis for the effective management of the illness was reflected in the sharp increase in home and life-cycle issues

[4] This interaction involving nurse, physician and social worker illustrates Thompson and McEwen's description of a coalition pursuing "a goal calling for more support, especially for more resources, than any one of them is able to marshall unaided." Cf. J. D. Thompson and W. McEwen, "Organizational Goals and Environment," *American Sociological Review*, XXIII (February, 1958), pp. 23-31.

addressed in the clinic (reflected by a rise from 13% to 31% in interaction involving this scope of content). The trend in home focused issues was particularly notable in waiting room contacts (shown by an increase from 9% to 24% in home and life cycle content of interaction there). The support that was the focus of help provided to this family was thus in line with the new community-oriented health care that was adopted in the clinic (Cf. Appendix B, Tables Ia, and Ib).

V-7. Home Issues and Community Health Services

The new community orientation adopted in the diabetic clinic also embraced more active contacts with health services in family communities. These contacts included close working relationships with visiting nurses associations and school health departments. They included sharing of information and planning of home visits. Discussions also focused prominently on relationships within families. The narrow technical focus which had been featured by the health teaching during the first year, gave way to a broader scope that included the social dimensions of family living.

V-8. Part-Time Clinic Structure and Community Orientation

The community orientation to diabetic health care was adopted in response to real organizational difficulties of the clinic. The diabetic services of the outpatient department were restricted to one afternoon session a week. During the remainder of the time physicians and nurses were not readily available. The clinic nurse, who spent the majority of her time in the surgical department, attempted to encourage families to phone her at the hospital if need should arise during the course of the week. Families frequently complained about the inadequacy of this arrangement. The head nurse took frequent occasion, in discussion with physicians and other staff members, to complain about the state of the hospital diabetic services. These complaints included pleas for full-time nursing personnel and the need to upgrade the quality of diabetic care provided by physicians. While requests for increase in nursing staff received open support from physicians and other staff personnel,[5] criticism of medical practice evoked ambiguous response.

[5] The structural weakness of the diabetic clinic was associated with continued supervisory control of physicians over nursing. Thus in addition to predictability of technology and professionalization as suggested by Bell, political factors influence supervisory control over discretionary personnel. Cf. G. Bell, "Formality versus Flexibility in Complex Organizations" in G. Bell, *Organizations and Human Behavior*, Englewood Cliffs, N. J.: Prentice-Hall, 1967, pp. 97-106.

In a structural context, the organizational rationale for the new community orientation is clarified. With the move, the status of the diabetic clinic declined. Few new resources were made available compared to those gained by the orthopedic and arthritis services. Small interest was displayed by the hospital toward diabetes as an area of research or toward stimulating diabetic medical practice.

In these circumstances, the effort to maintain the health teaching emphasis which marked the first year became unrealistic. The nursing department, working in collaboration with staff physicians, took the initiative in making contact with the social service department.[6] With the help of social workers as liaison persons, relationships were established with health resources in the home community.[7]

V-9. Organizational Discrepancy and Positive Adaptation to Change

The diabetes and arthritis services are examples of discrepant organizational units. In the arthritis department high political power in the hospital was combined with low technical control over the illness. With the move to the new building this organizational discrepancy created a power vacuum which was effectively exploited by the nursing department during examination room contacts with families.

In diabetes an opposite sort of organizational discrepancy existed, and was aggravated by the move to the new clinic. Political power within the hospital became further weakened[8] while technical control,

[6] Greater cooperation between health team specialists suggests the prescription of Dayal and Thomas for organizational success. In line with systems theory, these authors define organizational maturity as the simultaneous "differentiation" and "integration" of skills. Cf. I. Dayal and J. M. Thomas, "Operation KPE: Developing a New Organization," *Journal of Applied Behavioral Science,* IV (October-December, 1968), pp. 473-506.

[7] The combining processes involving nursing, physicians and social service in the hospital with health resources in the community illustrate a distinct feature of an organic system as specified by Burns and Stalker. Cf. T. Burns and E. M. Stalker, *The Management of Innovation,* London: The Tavistock Publications, 1961.

[8] The weakening of diabetes relative to surgery was partly a function of the supervision exercised over residents as pointed out by Nathanson. The focus of supervision was disease-oriented, which downgraded diabetes as a "garden-variety illness" as compared with the range of physical problems found in the surgical clinics. Cf. C. Nathanson, "Surveillance and Patient Orientation in a Pediatric Out-Patient Clinic," *Human Organization,* XXX (Fall, 1971), pp. 225-265. For a related discussion of problems of medical supervision relating to the issues of autonomy, professionalism and specialization, see the work of Freidson and Rhea. Cf. Eliot Freidson and Buford Rhea, "Processes of Control in a Company of Equals," *Social Problems,* XI (Fall, 1963), pp. 119-131; and Eliot Freidson and Buford Rhea, "Knowledge and Judgement in Professional Evaluations," *Administrative Science Quarterly,* X (June, 1965), pp. 107-124.

being high, provided opportunities for alternate paths for health service within home communities.[9] The nursing service was able to exploit a weak power position within the hospital by building bridges, through the social service department, to the homes and schools of children attending the clinic.[10] Although evidence of the effectiveness of this exploitation of weakness was not as firm as in arthritis, the data as derived from analysis of the tape recordings appears to support this conclusion (this evidence was supported by responses from home interviews with diabetic families).[11]

V-10. Increased Improvisation: Area Usage and Home Scope

A computer analysis of the coded data indicates the increased articulation of the diabetic clinic as a family based improvising system. Thus continued high level use of the waiting room (comprising 56% as compared with 57% of family contact for the previous year's observations) marked the persistence of the family orientation of the clinc.[12] At the same time, sharp increases were noted in the incidence of home and life cycle scope issues during family contacts. Home-related problems, as the content of waiting room interaction, rose in volume from 15.6% to 35.5% and staff initiation of home scope issues there augmented from 50.7% to 64.0%. At the same time there was an acceleration of the amount of non-medically related matter during examination room activities.[13]

A reversal occurred in the pattern of family and staff initiative in the separate cure and care centers of the clinic. Families showed a substantial increase in home-related problem initative during examination room contacts (from 24.4% to 61.5%). Staff showed a surge in initiative

[9] Jacques observed that individuals' ability to stand uncertainty and ambiguity governs the scope of the responsibility that will be sought. The present research suggests that uncertainty and ambiguity train individuals to seek responsibility. Cf. E. Jacques *The Measurement of Responsibility,* London: Tavistock Publications, 1956, pp. 85-106.

[10] Nursing relations with social service and community agencies to contact families in their homes illustrate Mechanic's observation that lower participants achieve control in complex organizations by circumventing rather than by using the role structure. The passive cooperation of physicians in the new community orientation suggests that power was achieved partly by circumventing the medical hierarchy. Cf. D. Mechanic, "Sources of power of lower participants in complex organizations," *Administrative Science Quarterly,* VII (December, 1962), p. 349.

[11] Questions raised with families relating to the quality of health services are contained in the Home Interview Questionnaire, Appendix C.

[12] Cf. Appendix B, Table Ib.

[13] Based on frequencies and percentages given in Table II, Appendix B. (Percentages given in Table II are for family initiation, while frequencies are for both family and staff initiative.)

regarding family problems in the waiting room area (from 50.7% to 64.0%).[14] This pattern of change suggested a redefinition of clinic areas during staff-family interaction. Families were much more able to use staff-related areas to discuss family issues, while staff members were much freer than before in discussing home focused issues in the family area of the waiting room. This greater flexibility in crossing institutionally symbolic boundaries was associated with improvisation within the clinic system.[15]

With a striking advance in home and life-cycle content the diabetic clinic showed a definite positive trend as an improvising system. Thus home and long-term life issues increased noticeably (from 13% to 31%), while medical and technical hospital problems declined sharply (from 87% to 69%) during overall clinic family interaction.[16] This was the most dramatic change in problem content in the course of the move of the outpatient department, and marked a trend toward intensified patterns of improvisation.[17] This tendency was in line with the new community orientation.

V-11. Community Orientation and Affective Channelling

In the first year's activities a strong affective trend had been observed. This tendency was associated with the prominence given to the autonomy training of children in the waiting room. The support structure provided by staff members and by families gathered there made possible diffuse patterns of social interaction. This diffusion appeared appropriately geared to the attempt to elicit from children and their families an active response in the management of the illness.

With the shift toward community orientation a change in affective patterning occurred. The emphasis moved from short-term goals sought through health teaching in the clinic to long-term planning in collaboration with social service and community agencies. This policy

[14] Based on family initiative percentages shown in Table II, Appendix B.

[15] To the extent to which families and staff were able to transcend institutional barriers during communication Thompson's model of heuristic-optional interaction was observed. Thus, diabetic nursing dealt with home issues in an "out-put role" with "reciprocating" families within a "transaction structure". Consistent with this transactional pattern home related issues met three distinguishable outcomes: "completion, abortion and side transactions." Cf. James D. Thompson, "Organizations and Output Transactions," *American Journal of Sociology,* LXVIII (November, 1962), pp. 300-324.

[16] Cf. Appendix B, Table Ia.

[17] This intensified improvisation signalled by greater attention to home-related problems is consistent with Buckley's analysis of "change of goal parameters" as a dimension of "feedback control of social goal seeking." Cf. Buckley, *Sociology and Modern Systems Theory,* pp. 172ff.

GRAPH K-V-11

Changes in Components of Affective Behavior in the Diabetes Clinic

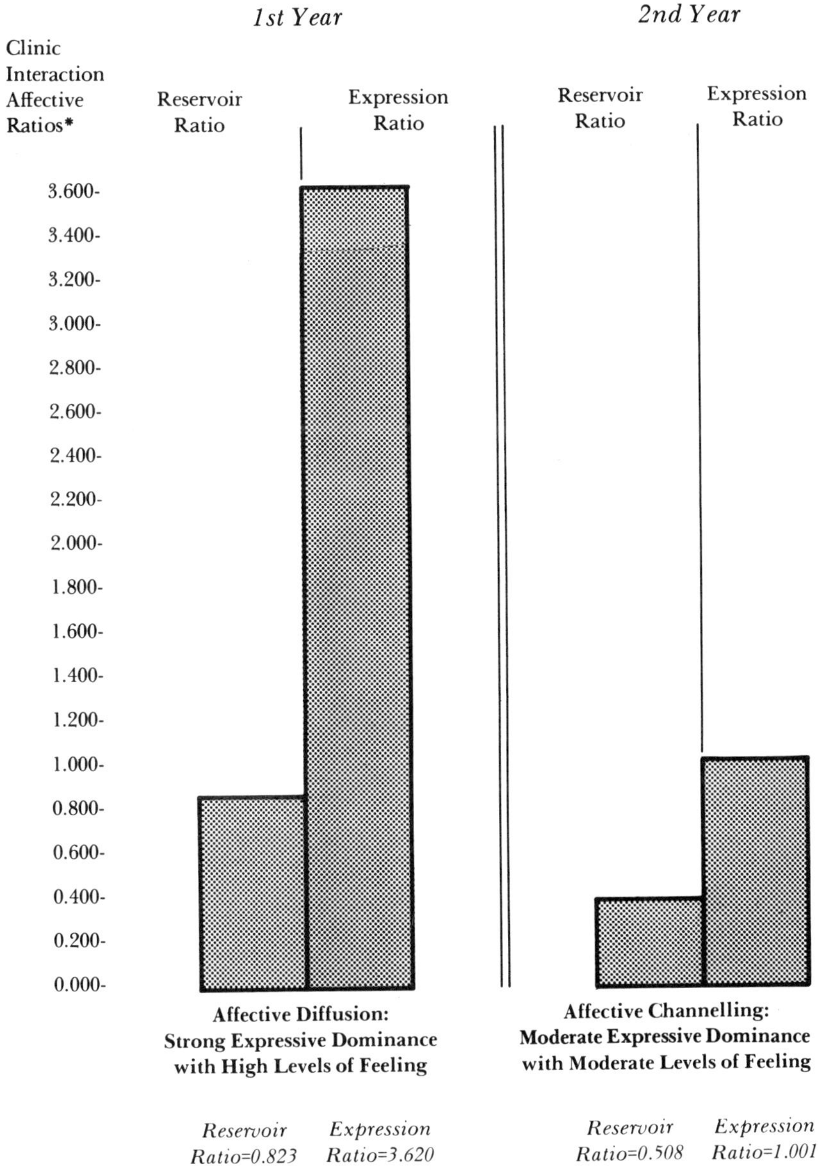

**Based on ratios presented in Table VII, Appendix B, p. 207.*

called for a more subdued approach during family contacts. The more muted toning was reflected in lower levels of feeling both during task activities and social sequences.[18]

The relatively narrower range of feeling levels between work and rest situations was associated with the discontinuance of intense autonomy teaching. A moderate but distinct rise in feelings connected with intensified work activities suggested a channelled approach to families in attempts to interest them in community health resources. This moderate fluctuation in the use of feelings during home-related problem discussion indicated a channelling of affect in the service of long-term objectives in the community. It contrasted with the diffuse patterns of extreme affective variation associated with efforts to achieve immediate results through autonomy teaching.[19]

The sharp contrast in emotional patterning from the previous year is shown in Graph K-V-11. While levels of feelings were sharply reduced, a moderate expressive dominance was maintained consistent with an affective channelling pattern.

V-12. Community Orientation and Unstructured Roles

Connected with the previous year's health teaching was a moderately high degree of interactive structuring. Staff members entered into interviews with a well-defined program of medically related matters to discuss. The focus was the children's management of diabetic care routines. With the new emphasis on collaboration with community services, a broader range of topics emerged. These embraced a wider range of home related issues in which families took noticeably greater initiative. The rigid role structuring (staff initiation of courtship and seek-

[18] Thus reserved feeling put forth in the absence of task objectives declined (from a reservoir ratio of 0.823 to 0.508), while expressed feelings employed during work sequences fell more abruptly (from an expression ratio of 3.620 to 1.1001.) An initial sharp expressive predominance (of +2.797) was reduced to a moderate expressive bias (of +0.493). This pattern while suggesting control of feelings, indicated a trend toward affective channelling. Cf. Appendix B, Table VII, Cols. 3, 4 and 5.

[19] This shift of the diabetic clinic toward affective channelling and use of community health resources is in line with Deutsch's analysis of a "learning net." Such a "learning net" is identified by the capacity of its constituent parts for regrouping themselves into new patterns of activity in response to changes in the net's surroundings or in response to internally accumulating changes within the net. K. W. Deutsch "Toward a Cybernetic Model of Man and Society," in Buckley, ed., *Modern Systems Research for the Behavioral Scientist,* p. 398.

ing of feedback; family specialization in small talk and feedback) toned down noticeably.[20]

This reduction of rigidity in interactive roles was especially strong in home scope problems. The overall differences in the expected clinic patterning of the four feedback-related variables decline noticeably when staff and family initiation are compared.[21]

Declines in structured role patterning were also evident in medical scope issues.[22] As shown in Graph L-V-12 the sharp earlier tendency for families to provide medical scope feedback and for staff to seek information on medical matters was noticeably reduced in the clinic.

These shifts indicated that with the new community-orientation, families assumed a more active posture toward staff, while interactive role assignment became more flexible.

V-13. Increased Interactive Improvisation and Feedback Responsiveness

A general trend toward greater improvisation evolved in the new diabetic clinic. That improvising patterns became strengthened is shown by increases in home-related concerns, greater family initiative and a decline in interactive role structuring. The declines noted in affective behavior resulted from a shift from a diffuse health teaching to a more channelled long-term collaboration with the home community.

A notable augmentation of responsiveness during feedback activities was associated with this cooperative and improvising interactive process. During the first year, the diabetic clinic was marked by the lowest level of feedback response observed in the course of the research.[23] With the move to the new clinic, the diabetic services showed the greatest increase in average family-staff feedback responsiveness attained by any of the clinics (from 16.2% to 26.1%). It was particularly interesting that this increase was largely due to greater activity on the part of families (family feedback response increased from 13.8% to 27.7% while

[20] The channelling of feeling and decline of role structure was in line with the description of the clinic as a destructurated network. Cf. F. D. Powell, "A Concept of Structurated and Destructurated Group Roles: An Initial Empirical Reduction." *Social Science and Medicine,* IV (September, 1970), pp. 321-327.

[21] Shown by an overall correlation change from 2.075 to 1.417, or 31.7%, in role patterning. Cf. Appendix B, Table V.

[22] Indicated by a correlation decrease in family versus staff initiation of +13.4% in role pattern difference. Cf. Appendix B, Table V, showing a decline in role structuring from 1.603 to 1.388.

[23] Indicated by an unweighted average unique response variance of 16.2% for staff and families. Cf. Appendix B, Table VI.

GRAPH L-V-12

Changes in Role Structuring in the Diabetic Clinic
(medical scope interaction*)

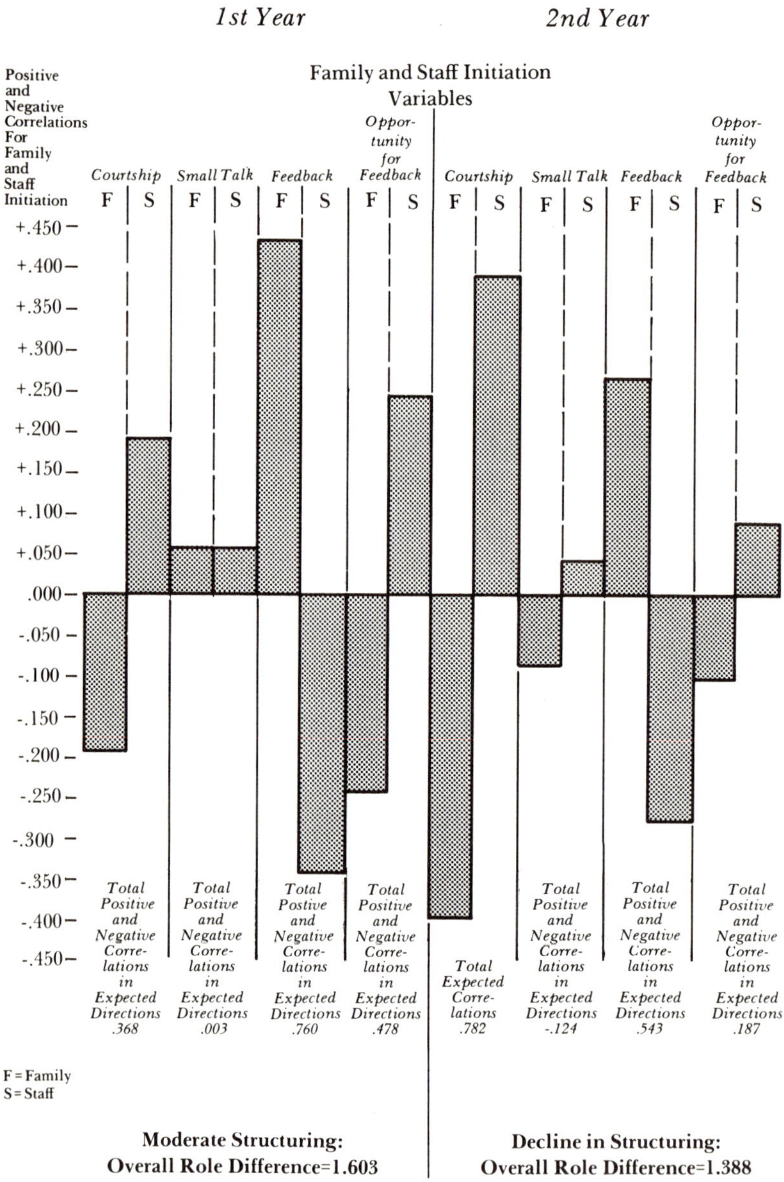

**Based on lagged correlations as presented in Table V, Appendix B, p. 206.*

staff response rose moderately from 18.5% to 24.4%). As shown in Graph M-V-13 feedback process evolved from a low to a moderately high response pattern, while staff dominance was replaced by family dominance.

A similar rise in family feedback responsiveness in arthritis (from 6.7% to 21.0%) suggested that in both clinics increases in improvising interaction were associated with more responsive feedback processes.[24]

[24] This rise in feedback effectiveness in both clinics was associated with greater awareness of long-term time perspectives and is thus consistent with a "true feedback" approach suggested by Buckley. Cf. Buckley *Sociology and Modern Systems Theory,* pp. 172ff.

GRAPH M-V-13

Change in Feedback Responsiveness by Families and Staff in the Diabetes Clinic

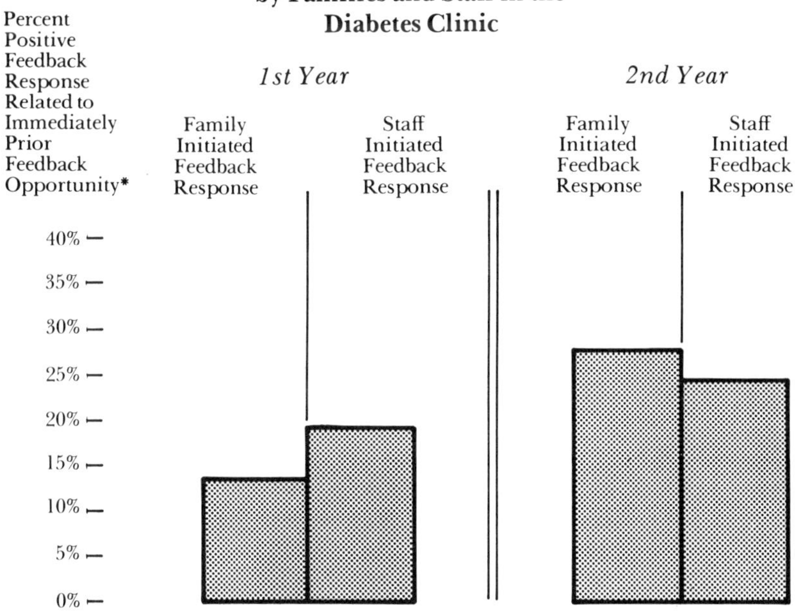

Low Overall Response with Moderate Staff Dominance
Average (unweighted) Family-Staff Feedback Response=16.2%
Specific Feedback Response
Family=13.8%
Staff=18.5%

Moderately High Overall Response with Slight Family Dominance
Average (unweighted) Family-Staff Feedback Response=26.1%
Specific Feedback Response
Family=27.7%
Staff=24.4%

**Based on lagged regression analysis of data presented in Table VI, Appendix B, p. 207.*

V-14. Positive Change in a Family Based Improvising Organization

Positive trends observed in the diabetic services viewed as a family based improvising system were related to the increased institutional discrepancy of the clinic within the hospital structure. The further weakening of the political power of diabetes in the hospital presented the opportunity for non-autonomous professionals including nurses and social workers to explore alternate effective medical resources. The inability of the clinic to sustain an autonomy health teaching program opened up the opportunity to exploit community health and social service options. With the cooperation of a weakened staff of physicians, the nursing department instituted ties with social workers and nurses in the hospital and within home communities.[25]

The development of this community health program led to increased articulation of the clinic as a family-based improvising system.[26] Use of the waiting room as a family-based care center continued, with renewed emphasis on home-related problems. Similar trends in examination room interaction marked the new clinic as a polycentered home-oriented service. Further improvisation was indicated by increased role flexibility and family initiative. These tendencies toward higher levels of improvising interaction were closely related to greater sensitivity in the clinic as judged through feedback responsiveness.[27]

These quantitative observations substantiate qualitative judgments

[25] The strategy and tactics followed in the arthritis and diabetic clinics relate to the "strong man" and "weak man" bargaining behavior suggested by Psathas and Stryker. Thus in arthritis where there was a discrepancy between the level of power (high) and the level of technology (low) an increase in political status led to a "strong man" strategy of occupancy of the power area and intensified improvisation tactics with families. In diabetes a reduced political position induced a "weak man" strategy of use of interstitial areas for coalitions with social service and visiting nurses to exploit alternate effective community technical resources. Cf. Psathas and Stryker, "Bargaining Behavior and Orientations in Coalition Formation," *Sociometry* XXVIII (June, 1965), pp. 124-144. The diabetic response also suggests a high productive affiliation arousal pattern. Cf. R. De Charms, "Affiliation Motivation and Productivity in Small Groups," *Journal of Abnormal and Social Psychology,* LV (1957), pp. 222-26. Cf. D. C. McClelland, *The Achieving Society,* New York: Collier-Macmillan, 1968.

[26] Perrow in describing task structures ascribes intensive feedback activities to flexible, polycentralized systems. This description applies to the new diabetes services. Cf. C. Perrow, "A Framework for the Comparative Analysis of Organizations," *American Sociological Review,* XXXII (April, 1967), pp. 194-208.

[27] These positive trends in improvisation are consistent with the analysis of the clinic as a destructurated network. Nursing staff exploitation of institu-

of health services provided to families. Despite complaints about the grade of diabetic care, the new diabetic clinic displayed more capacity to deal with the individual needs of families, especially those related to the home environment. There was moreover a definite increase in the ability to exploit realistically the health resources inside and outside the hospital.

The exploitation of these resources was generated, as in the arthritis clinic, by institutional discrepancy.[28] A deterioration of the already weak hospital political base enabled nurses and social workers to exploit effective community health options. Successful pursuit of these alternatives led to positive change within the clinic; a change which brought about increased sensitivity of the clinic, as a system providing support to families coping with the problems of diabetic children.

tional discrepancies, and collaboration with social service and community agencies manifested positive feedback and interpenetration of roles. Cf. F. D. Powell, "A Concept of Structurated and Destructurated Group Roles," *Social Science and Medicine,* IV (September, 1970), p. 122.

[28] These innovations resemble the "unplanned institutional development" which Clark found to be a factor of "decentralization." "Greater leeway for initiative and innovation" by "subordinate personnel" and by "field administrators" parallels the collaboration of nursing and social service in diabetes with community health services. The "decentralization" of the diabetic clinic relative to the surgical power structure, facilitated the exploitation of political weakness by these "subordinate personnel." Cf. B. Clark, *Adult Education in Transition: A Study of Institutional Insecurity,* Berkeley: University of California Press, 1968, especially pp. 85, 106-7 and 150.

CHAPTER VI

THE ORTHOPEDIC CLINIC: A STAFF BASED RITUAL ORGANIZATION

The orthopedic clinic displayed some characteristics of a crisis unit.[1] Despite certain crisis qualities, however, the clinic manifested coping characteristics with staff-based and ritual dimensions. The presence of a substantial number of children with long-range bone correction problems, raised the issue of the child's basic body image and was a source of anxiety to families and staff. Such was the case particularly with families having children suffering from scoliosis, a condition forcing serious spinal surgery with possible life-long physical handicaps. Efforts by the staff to establish routine relationships with families sprang from a desire to minimize concern for these long-range effects, and to defend against anxieties related to the issue of body image.

These efforts to minimize and defend against anxiety were highlights of the clinic. Examination rooms were used rather than public

[1] Crisis units, such as fire departments, police squads, undertaking establishments, and emergency units of general hospitals, are distinguished from coping systems by their designed responsibility for short-run stressful situations. Cf. M. Lefton and W. R. Rosengren, "Organizations and Clients: Lateral and Longitudinal Dimensions," *American Sociological Review,* XXXI (Dec., 1966), for a schematic analysis of crisis units.

areas for family contact, as an institutionalized locational strategy.[2] This strategic approach was complemented by ritualized, tactical elements of low expressiveness, a moderate degree of structuring, and tendencies to emphasize medical scope and staff initiative. The direction of parents and children through the hospital bureaucracy was an important part of the orthopedic nursing service. This evoked a lively feedback responsiveness between families and staff.

VI-1. Organization of the Clinic

During the two years of activities in the orthopedic clinic, interaction was recorded with over two hundred families, ninety of whom attended the first year's sessions. Many of the children had foot and leg problems which were correctable within periods of from six months to two years, but a substantial number of cases involved more complex difficulties calling for surgery and lengthy periods of bone correction using casts and braces.

Important differences existed between the orthopedic and arthritis clinics as surgical services due to the size of the clinics and the chronicity of the conditions treated. The small size of the arthritis clinic and the chronic nature of the condition led to a degree of intimacy and personal relation with families. A key factor in the quality of the service in arthritis was the use of clinic notes in preparation for family conferences. These interviews were much more individualized in a small clinic with relatively few patients returning often to see the same staff members.

The atmosphere of the orthopedic clinic was rather impersonal and fast moving; it was not unusual for as many as fifty or sixty families to be seen on a single day. Continued contact between particular families and clinic staff was not usual, and careful preparation of cases and individualized care of families was usually not attempted. Physicians and nurses appeared to give less attention to families and tried to define the children's condition as routine in character.

VI-2. Physical Make-Up of the Clinic

The emotional distance which characterized the clinic was accentuated by its physical organization. The facilities consisted of a rather small waiting room, thirty by twenty-five feet, with three adjacent examina-

[2] Cf. F. D. Powell, "A Concept of Structurated and Destructurated Group Roles," *Social Science and Medicine,* IV (September, 1970), pp. 321-227. See below also Appendix A, Methodology, A-5 and A-6, for a discussion of the conceptual dimensions of ritual patterns which tended to predominate during orthopedic interaction. Cf. above II-16, for related description of ritual and improvising interactive patterns.

tion rooms. In addition there was a laboratory and cast room, serviced by technical personnel. At the side of the waiting room was a small administration desk where the clinic clerk received families. Just off the waiting room was a small room hardly larger than a closet that was used by the staff nurse as an office. (See Figure B-III-1, p. 34 above.)

In these cramped quarters it was not uncommon to find thirty families, of two or three members each, crowding the clinic. In an effort to expand the orthopedic facilities the examination rooms were divided by curtains so that several patients and their families could be interviewed and examined by physicians at the same time, an unnecessary procedure during arthritis clinic hours.

During the first period of the research the staff nurse, who was also the head nurse in arthritis, was the only full time member of the clinic nursing staff. During an average day in the clinic four or five physicians were in attendance over a period of six or seven hours. Due to the large number of families and the shortage of examination rooms and staff, there was very little opportunity for close contacts with families.

VI-3. Clinic Leadership Problems

The absence of the chief of the clinic due to illness contributed to the emotional detachment and poor organization of the clinic during the first period of the research. Tardiness and non-appearance by physicians was criticized both by staff and families. Part of the nurses' duties was to confront irate parents, some of whom had to wait four or five hours in the reception area to see a physician. Out of this confusion and delay the head nurse emerged in the role of "traffic cop" and mediator between families, administrative staff and physicians in the conflicting demands for attention. As a matter of routine the nurse spent a great deal of her time checking the order of families awaiting appointments and assigning rooms to families, where they awaited the services of specific physicians.

The assignment of physicians to patients tended to be rather complicated and it frequently happened that the nurse had to make the decision. Usually she would inquire whether a family had seen a particular physician on previous visits to the clinic. If the family expressed a preference for a certain doctor the nurse would make an effort to obtain his services; however, in many cases the physician was absent or was no longer a member of the staff. In such cases it was the nurse who decided which physician the family would see.

The nurse frequently was also called upon to decide whether a family would be able to see any physician at all during a particular session. Due to the shortage of space and of staff doctors there was a strong inclination to give priority to patients who had accurate records and charts. In many cases the failure to locate the appropriate information in the outpatient record room led to the decision that the family would have to return another day. In such cases the nurse invariably would consult with a senior physician, and her recommendation would be followed.

The absence of the clinic chief increased the nurse's administrative role. Since interns and residents were usually busy with families it became her duty to select children for specialty clinics and to propose specific physicians for particular patients. Although such decisions were always discussed with staff doctors they appeared content to let the nurse assume this responsibility.

The administrative role of the orthopedic nurse was further emphasized by the absence of the regular clinic clerk. This accentuated her role as "traffic cop" (a title that was self-conferred) and as arbitrator of disputes with families. In this capacity the nurse carried on a constant struggle with the X-ray department and the record room in frequent and often unsuccessful efforts to obtain charts and information.[3]

VI-4. Preservation of Routine by Humor and Social Distance

The orthopedic clinic was a general surgical clinic oriented primarily to routine problems. When unusual cases arose there was a tendency for physicians and nurses either to ignore them or to minimize the problems.[4] Humor was a device for coping in a routine manner with stressful situations.[5] This is illustrated by an exchange with a four-year-old boy who attended the clinic with his aunt. The child had an ordinary foot problem that could readily be corrected by means of an orthopedic shoe. But there was clear indication of emotional complications suggested by his recent refusal to walk. This behavior upset the mother who called the aunt. The latter with some effort finally persuaded the child to walk. The fact that the aunt brought the child in rather than the mother, suggested the possibility of a disturbed family pattern. The observer noted the failure of either the physician or the nurse to obtain information or to refer the family to social services for follow-up.

[3] Thus a very high percentage of problems, namely 60%, were administrative in character in the orthopedic clinic. This compared with 22% in diabetic, 27% in cystic fibrosis and 52% in arthritis during the first year. (These figures are based on a hand-process analysis of the data.)

[4] Rosengren and De Vault speak of the use of specialized medical areas by staff to maintain "studied casualness" by means of "tempo, timing and rhythm." Cf. W. R. Rosengren and S. De Vault, "The Sociology of Time and Space in an Obstetrical Hospital," in E. Freidson, ed., *The Hospital in Modern Society*, especially pp. 278-285.

[5] Cf. Rosengren and De Vault for a parallel analysis of medical area behavior. *Ibid.*

The discussion with the family proceeded:

Aunt to physician: So I went over there, 'cos I had an automobile. . . . When I got there, he wouldn't get up to get it. And then, well, she said, "Come over and get it, Edward." And he wouldn't. So, well, okay, so I said, "Let me take your hand," and I walked him up and down for a few minutes.

Physician to aunt: Yes. He's a headstrong little fellow, is he?

Aunt to physician: Yes, that's when she decided it.

Physician to aunt *(laughing):* That's when she decided that he was, huh?

Aunt to physician: But, I mean, he's perfectly normal in his way.

Physician to aunt: Yes.

Aunt to physician: He's smart.

[At this point in the interaction the physician directed the young child to walk up and down, and having examined his feet and legs prescribed an orthopedic shoe as a correction. The interaction continued as follows.]

Physician to aunt: Yes. Now I've got you a prescription for him.

Aunt to physician: For another shoe?

Physician to aunt: Yes.

Aunt to physician: Oh good. And that's all it is?

Physician to aunt: Yep, that's all it is. His foot is fine, I'm sure.

Nurse to physician: Will you have him come back, Dr. Jones?

Physician to nurse: Yes.

Nurse to aunt: See, all set. . . . well, he just looks like a very active boy, but it's always [good] to check out any kind of . . .

Physician to aunt: Yes, we'll see him again in six months. If he should limp again or refuse to walk again in the meanwhile, well we ought to see him right away. But [it] sound[s] to me like this was more . . .

Aunt to physician *(interrupting):* . . . emotional.

Physician to aunt: Emotional, than physical.

Aunt to physician: I think it was, 'cos the child was all right afterwards, and he doesn't mix with his family or own relations, two brothers and a sister. But he mixes tremendously with the other kids that I bring him to. A lot of my friends have six or seven kids and he doesn't quarrel with them.

Physician to aunt: You have to mix there if you don't get run over.

Aunt to physician: I mean he's sharp.

Nurse to aunt: Survival of the fleetest.

Physician to aunt: That's right, the fleetest.

The physician and nurse systematically ignored the family's social and emotional problems. At no point did the nurse explore the reason the aunt rather than the mother brought the child to the clinic. Neither physician nor nurse commented on the fact that the child's behavior within the family seemed withdrawn, and the doctor attributed his refusal to walk to stubbornness.[6]

With this family, humor was used to minimize or deny the home problems involved. When informed that the child got along well with friends when away from his family, both physician and nurse dismissed the contrast with joking responses.[7]

This concern with preserving routine was partly the result of the administrative involvement of the nurse and the understaffing of medical personnel. The nurse complained that her constant employment as "traffic cop" and general troubleshooter for difficulties arising in the clinic prevented her from spending sufficient time with families, particularly in health teaching.[8] Nurses and physicians appeared constantly on their guard against becoming involved with complex issues in order to maintain the speed required to deal with the large number of families attending the clinic sessions.[9]

[6] The staff ignored the aunt's concern for the child's emotional problems, consonant with Roth's view of professional attempts to keep the relationship role-specific whereas client goals are more general. Cf. J. Roth, "The Treatment of Tuberculosis as a Bargaining Process," in A. Rose, *Human Behavior and Social Process,* Boston: Houghton Mifflin, 1962, p. 577.

[7] The use of humor to minimize social and emotional problems by nurse and physician during this interview illustrates staff proprietary rights in a group territory defined as permitting discussion only of medical issues. Cf. Goffman, *Asylums,* p. 239.

[8] This administrative absorption was indicated by a 44.8% of nursing time spent with staff members other than physicians while no family was present. This figure was higher than in any other clinic. A comparably low figure of 43.6% was recorded for contact with families. (These figures are based on a line count of the transcribed recordings.) Cf. Appendix B, Table X.

[9] A contrast in clinic attitudes was reflected by the fact that in arthritis activity emotional problems constituted 26% of issues discussed with families, whereas during that year only 14% of the difficulties dealt with in the ortho-

In comments to the observer, the nurse expressed her expectations for improved opportunity for health teaching in the new building. In the crowded conditions of the clinic, when confronted with emotionally charged problems, the nurse either used humor or turned to physicians as a means of escape from the situation. When issues arose for which there was not adequate time, she would frequently terminate discussion with the assurance that the physician would soon be there to assist the family.[10]

As a result, the emotional tone of interaction between staff and families was restrained. Thus, when courtship behavior by staff is compared with that in the diabetes clinic, orthopedics was noticeably lower, suggesting a great variation in social distance in the two services.[11]

VI-5. Staff Based Family Contact

The orthopedic clinic as a staff-based system employed the examination rooms and adjacent medical areas for 88% of staff contact with families.[12] Moreover, when areas of the hospital are ranked in terms of degrees of staff-related versus family-related character, the orthopedic clinic scored highest[13] of all the outpatient services in staff-based area usage.[14] Indeed, direct statements by the head nurse indicated that preference for the use of medical areas, especially the examination room, reflected a policy of the orthopedic staff.

pedic clinic were emotional in character. This contrast was even greater in respect to diabetes, where 37% of problems were of an emotional nature. (Figures based on hand processing of the data.)

[10] Cf. the work of Georges Gurvitch *(The Spectrum of Social Time,* trans. Myrtle Kovenbaum, Dordrecht: Reidel, 1964) for a conceptual approach to the time dimensions of social networks. Cf. also J. Roth, *Timetables; Structuring the passage of time in hospital treatment and other careers,* Indianapolis: Bobbs-Merrill, 1963, for a parallel treatment of differences in time perspective between staff and family.

[11] Thus "courtship" initiated by staff was 1.933 in orthopedic in the first year in contrast during the same time period with a mean of 3.300 in diabetes. Cf. Appendix B, Tables XVIII and XIX. Figures are based on a five-point rating scale. Cf. Appendix, A-3 and A-4, for coding procedures regarding "courtship".

[12] This compared with family examination room contacts of 8% in cystic fibrosis, 35% in diabetes and 97% in arthritis. Cf. Table Ib, Appendix B.

[13] 4.23.

[14] The comparable scores for cystic fibrosis were 1.29, for diabetic, 2.44 and arthritis, 3.59. Excess of staff-based scores in orthopedic over arthritis resulted from use of the cast room and other back region medical locations.

A conversation between the nurse and a young assistant points up the policy for area usage:

Assistant to staff nurse: When there are two of us here in the general one, there will probably be a group in the waiting room teaching too?

Staff nurse to assistant: Oh, yes. This . . .

Assistant to staff nurse *(interrupting):* 'Cos parents then seem so warm and they [listen] to what you say, there's someone else that's just all ears.

Staff nurse to assistant: What kind of teaching do you think we need, general kinds of teaching or specific ones?

Assistant to staff nurse: Well, if you had all different kinds . . . if you had for instance several mothers with children with casts, if you could just talk to one about casts, they would all join in.

Staff nurse to assistant: They might.

Assistant to staff nurse: Well, it would rely, I think, as to whether the waiting room was made up of all different kinds of things which you would maybe then mean general teaching which is our job.

Staff nurse to assistant: [In the new building] there is a separate waiting room for the plaster patients and a separate waiting room for . . . the big general waiting room for the general patients. For instance, you might have all your mothers with babies with club foot casts on in one area where you could approach them.

Assistant to staff nurse: Yeah.

Staff nurse to assistant: You can do it to a degree. You can also run across many people who don't want to discuss things like this. Like I say the chronic problems are deformities as far as the parents are concerned and many of them prefer to have that door shut before they start to talk. And many of them will relate better to you if they think it's a personal thing between you and them. You might in some cases jeopardize this relationship by a general discussion. So that it depends on what it's about. On general health principles I think it's very good, very good, and on cast kids, but there are other things which . . . try it out. You will soon know. If the mother who is involved in a discussion out there, gets into a room and clams up, you'll know something is wrong. They're very private about some of their problems. I don't know if I like it.

The observer commented that the staff nurse's response was more indicative of the way the staff nurse "thinks about it than it is an objective answer." The import of this remark is underlined by a reflection by the observer that the staff nurse did not enter the waiting room during a whole week of clinic activities. In fact the nurse's use of the waiting room was extremely limited and brief. Periodically, she would appear in the waiting room, call to a family whose turn it was for an appointment, and escort them to an examination room, to be seen by a physician. Only 6% of family contacts occurred in the waiting room. This compared with frequencies of family waiting room contact of 87% in cystic fibrosis, 57% in diabetes, and only 2% in the arthritis clinic.[15]

Employment of the examination room as choice location for family conferences is reminiscent of patterns observed in the arthritis clinic. However, behavior in the two clinics suggests contrasting approaches to the use of the examination room. The comparison is of particular interest since the same nurse was involved in the two clinics. In the arthritis clinic the examination room was used by families to raise problems, frequently related to non-physical, home-related situations. One family chose the examination room to tell the nurse of publicity that the child had received from the local arthritis association. Another used the examination room to express emotional feelings that mother and child had had when a cast was first put on. Arthritis families also used the examination room to discuss school problems and occupational therapy. In the examination room with arthritis patients the nurse responded supportively to social and emotional issues initiated by families.

In the orthopedic clinic where the fast pace and crowded conditions of the clinic produced an air of impersonality, physicians and nurses used the examination room as an area of defense against feelings and social issues. In the case of the aunt and four-year-old boy, the fears of the aunt about emotional factors were denied by both physician and nurse. The situation provided by the examination room enabled the staff to define the situation in medical terms. Although in the conversation with the assistant the nurse insisted on the examination room as a choice location for establishing a relationship with families, the area was frequently employed to suit the limited medical perspective of staff members.[16]

[15] Cf. Appendix B, Table Ib.

[16] The narrow physical approach was reflected in the comparison of scope of problems dealt with in the examination room. In arthritis 44% of the issues were medical, while 53% were home related. In the orthopedic clinic, of the problems handled in the examination room, 53% were medical while 30% were home related. Cf. Appendix B, Table Ib.

VI-6. Dependency and Medical Scope of Treatment

The narrow medical approach stressing physical aspects of the illness was related to a tendency to emphasize the dependency of families on the medical system. These patterns were illustrated by further remarks of the staff nurse to the assistant about another family which had been visiting the clinic over some period of time. The discussion pertained to a father, a mother and two children, the older a boy aged three, who was suffering from a serious partially uncorrectable hip condition.

> **Staff nurse to nursing assistant:** He came along and every time we tried to relocate his hips, it seemed we broke a leg, because he had such . . . but he's never stood up, he's never been on his feet at all. And so to one fracture after the other, and doing his exercises he'll get the buckle fracture and, oh, it was just terrible and she just went through hell. Back and forth to the hospital, and her entire life was wrapped around this kid. The brand new husband of one year just sort of sat in the background from the beginning. So it was a very unusual family, very odd and very unhealthy family situation. Then she lost a pregnancy, sure, when she lost it, that it was abnormal like this one. She became pregnant a third time, and delivered a healthy, normal baby, who is now, well, I would hazard a guess at six or eight months old. And he's okay. Well, she still spends all her time with this one. When she has the physical therapist going at home, she has lots of reassurance, she can do things herself, but she won't do them, she needs help. She is very dependent, and she gets very irate easily at the stubborn child, like an 18-year-old or a 16-year-old. And she does it when things don't quite go her way. She's paying money now for a baby sitter, that she really can't afford to pay. Now why the dickens, if I may use that word, they aren't concerned with the future of the kids, I don't know. It would seem more reasonable, but I'm not going to go into that, [it's] not that much my business. But when she gives me the business, I just give it back to her. With this kind of person you have to, because she has to be treated like a teenager, because she behaves like one. And she'll just go back, she'll sulk a little while, then she'll be all right, but she'll always come back to me again for help. But if I just, you know, ignored her or gave in to her or something like that, I don't think she would. So you have to really maintain a firm hand with her.

The nursing assistant, in talking with this mother had found that the immediate medical problem stemmed from the child's difficulty in being put on his stomach while in traction. The assistant said to the staff nurse that the child would scream and refuse to cooperate and that the problem lay in the mother's inability to maintain her authority with the child in the management of the treatment. The difficulties were further complicated by the unwillingness of the father to become involved.

It is of interest to note that about twenty-five minutes were spent by the staff nurse explaining to this mother the correct procedures in the preparation of sterile bandages to be applied to the hip of the child. The time spent on the physical management of the illness was in sharp contrast with the lack of attention to dependency and planning. While recognizing the parents' inability to deal with the behavior of the children, the nurse asserted that she could not become involved. Toward the immaturity of the mother, the nurse adopted a policy of firmness and used the mother's dependency to insure that she would return to the clinic for help.[17]

The nurse's attitude was that future problems were no concern of the clinic. This attitude was in sharp contrast with that in the arthritis clinic where the same nurse was involved. There, in dealing with chronic problems, efforts were made to provide opportunities for occupational therapy and to help patients accept the long-term character of the illness.[18]

The disparity in response of the nurse is most revealing of the vast differences between the arthritis and orthopedic clinics. The *same* nurse operating in the *same* location displayed such polarity in her behavior that the staffing and operational difficulties of the orthopedic clinic are dramatically brought out.

The response to home-related and life cycle goals in the arthritis clinic stand in sharp contrast with the attitude in the orthopedic clinic. The nurse manipulated the dependency of the mother in order to make sure that she continued to return to the clinic.[19] The fact that by so

[17] The disapprobation and narrow medical approach adopted toward this family supports the view that outpatient staff tend to regard as "good patients" those who follow routines. Cf. A. O. Playa, L. M. Cohen, & J. Samora, "Communication between Physicians and Patients in Out Patient Clinics: Social and Cultural Factors," *Millbank Foundation Quarterly,* April, 1968, Vol. 46, No. 2, part 1, pp. 161-213.

[18] The contrast in behavior between the two clinics underlines the "importance of amenities" suggested by Freidson in reaffirming the patient's dignity and in initiating a social relationship encouraging cooperation in treatment. Cf. E. Freidson, "Organizing Ambulatory Care," in *Professional Dominance: The Social Structure of Medical Care,* New York: Atherton Press, 1970, p. 197.

[19] The tendency toward "primitive trust" or simple dependency on the staff is reflected in the handling of the problems of this family. The emphasis on a more "mature trust" in the arthritis clinic may be inferred from the greater attention given there to home and life cycle scope problems. For comparison

doing she might increase the problems of the family and in the long run complicate the difficulties of the mother in coping with the physical problems of a rebellious child was considered beyond the scope of the clinic. Such problems presumably would be met episodically as they arose.

VI-7. Avoidance of Children

There was marked tendency in the orthopedic clinic for communication from the nurse to be directed to the parents rather than to the child. The nurse initiated with parents 50.1% of the interaction with families, while only 12.5% of nursing initiation was with children. Parents initiated 33.5% of the interaction with the nurse, while children's responses to the staff constituted only 3.9% of the communication.[20]

This contrasted with the diabetic clinic where 25.5% of staff communication was directed to parents, while 40.8% was intended for the child. Also in diabetes parents were somewhat more active relative to the nurse (23.0% of initiation as compared with 25.5% nurse to parent initiative).[21]

The tendency to avoid communication with children in the orthopedic clinic, as compared with diabetes, can be partly accounted for by differences in the nature of the illnesses. The need for the inculation of autonomy on the part of patients in diabetes accounted for the large percentage of communication directed to children.

VI-8. Anxiety as a Factor in Avoidance of Children

There was, however, an additional factor in the tendency of the staff to address parents rather than the child. Although orthopedic conditions encountered were usually short term in nature, and could frequently be cured by relatively routine medical procedures, there was an undertone of anxiety between staff and families not present in some of the other clinics. This sense of apprehension was traceable to the character of the condition being treated. In the orthopedic clinic, even though conditions were relatively routine from a medical point of view, there was a prominent degree of fear manifested by parents. With a mother concerned about her child's minor foot problem the nurse addressed

of scope of problems in the two clinics, cf. Appendix B, Table Ia, p. 201. For discussion of "mature trust" cf. E. H. Erikson, *Identity and the Life Cycle in Psychological Issues,* Vol. I, no. 1, New York: International Universities Press, 1959.

[20] Cf. Appendix B, Table XIII.

[21] Cf. Appendix B, Table XII.

herself directly to this anxiety and appeared to have been successful in reducing her fears. The mother's anxiety was related to the issue of body image.

Problems in orthopedics, however routine medically, involve family anxieties about specific body image concerns for the child. In dealing with this concern the nurse tried to convince mothers that the bone structure problems of the children were correctable. By developing trust in the effectiveness of medicine to cure the condition, the nurse seemed to be trying to overcome specific body image fears of parents.

There was usually some temporary imperfection in the child's bone structure, and often some uncertainty as to whether it could be corrected. There was thus a tendency to avoid reference to the child as a potential threat to the trust in orthopedic medicine that the nurse was trying to instill.

The presence of the child in the situation was a source of double anxiety to the nurse. She dealt with this anxiety through avoidance and directed her communication largely to the mother even when his age suggested that the child be included in the discussion. This avoidance behavior was also prominent at the end of interviews when the nurse often used humor at the expense of the child. Such sallies by the nurse seemed to be attempts to relax her own tension, and were, perhaps, an unconscious wish that the child were not present to threaten the trust and feeling of normalcy she was attempting to convey to the mother. The presence of the child was a threat to the nurse's trust in the power of medicine, and disturbing to the content of communication with the mother.

This interpretation derives support from data gleaned from observation in the arthritis clinic. Of all interaction between nurse and arthritis family members, 51.4% was initiated by the parents compared with only 41.1% initiated by the nurse. But only 6.9% involved initiation by the nurse to the child while merely 0.6% was initiated by children themselves.[22] This indicated a higher degree of avoidance of children than in the orthopedic clinic. This was noteworthy since the children attending the arthritis clinic were older than those in orthopedics.[23]

Insofar as immobility of the joints is a problem in the illness, the issue of body image was also present in arthritis. Since the problem was regarded as chronic, and the illness not considered curable, the anxiety of staff and parents was higher than in orthopedics. This resulted in a tendency of nurse and parents to avoid communication

[22] Cf. Appendix B, Table XI.

[23] The average age of children visiting the two services was 7.2 years in arthritis and 5.2 years in the orthopedic clinic.

with the child. This avoidance is highlighted by the fact that in the first year's observation, out of 2,320 words spoken between staff and families in arthritis only 13 were spoken by children.

VI-9. Authority and Pronoun Reference to Physicians

The large number of patients at sessions of the orthopedic clinic, many of whom had no previous contact with the staff, gave an atmosphere of impersonality to the setting. The shortage of staff and limitations of space led to long periods of waiting and to impatience. These conditions contributed an authoritarian character to the setting. Families attending the clinic displayed isolated, withdrawn and dependent patterns of behavior. Occasionally individuals would react to their frustration by expressing themselves aggressively. This resulted in conflict with clerical staff, nurses and physicians, about the time of appointments for their children. In this confused situation there was a tendency for nurses, clinic staff and family members to refer to physicians as authority figures.

The psychological issue of trust was also related to the importance given to physicians in the clinic. The physician as a symbol of the power of medicine was prominently mentioned in dialogues between nurses and parents. By contrast, in the other clinics such as diabetes and cystic fibrosis, where the issue of physician trust was not so relevant to treatment, fewer references to doctors were made.

A tabulation was made of third person pronoun references[24] to physicians when only nurses and families were present in clinic interactions. Orthopedic physicians were referred to in the third person at a rate of once every 21.1 lines of interaction.[25] This compared with a rate of once every 31.4 lines in arthritis. The frequency in the diabetic clinic was once in every 39.7 lines, while in cystic fibrosis physicians were

[24] Works dealing with theory and methods of sociolinguistics, and the related fields of ethnomethodology and phenomenology, include: Stephen Tyler, *Cognitive Anthropology,* New York: Holt, Rinehart and Winston, 1969; John Agar, *Ripping and Running,* New York: Seminar Press, 1973; John Gumperz and Dill Hyman, *New Directions in Sociolinguistics,* New York: Holt, Rinehart and Winston, 1971; Alfred Schutz, *Alfred Schutz on Phenomenology and Social Relations,* edited by Helmut R. Wagner, Heritage of Sociology Series, Chicago: University of Chicago Press, 1970; Alfred Schutz, *The Problem of Social Reality,* Vol. I, edited by M. Natanson, *Studies in Social Theory,* Vol. II, edited by A. Broderson, *Studies in Phenomenological Philosophy,* Vol. III, edited by A. Gurvitsch, *Collected Papers,* New York: Humanities Press, Inc., 1962-1966; Alfred Schutz, *Phenomenology of the Social World,* translated by G. Walsh and F. Lehnert (Studies in Phenomenology and Existential Philosophy Set), Evanston, Ill.: Northwestern University Press, 1967.

[25] Cf. Appendix B, Table XIV, Col. 4.

referred to on the average of once in every 383.2 lines. These differences between the four clinics reflect the degree to which trust in physicians was stressed in the treatment process.[26]

VI-10. Social Isolation and Non-Use of Collective Pronouns

A parallel and almost inverse order between the clinics was observed in the use of first person plural pronouns by mothers. This was used as an indication of the social isolation experienced by family members attending the clinic. It is assumed that the more this collective form of expression was employed the less the sense of social isolation on the part of families.

This collective expression was employed in the orthopedic clinic once in every 118 lines.[27] In the diabetic clinic the figure was once for every 74 lines, while the average in cystic fibrosis was one time for every 30 lines of initiation. These frequencies suggest that the greatest sense of social isolation was experienced in the orthopedic clinic. On the other hand, in arthritis, where the same nurse was involved, such collective expression occurred once in every 53 lines. The more frequent use of collective expression by families in arthritis as compared with that in the orthopedic clinic was related to a differential concern with long-range problems. In the highly bureaucratic and impersonal setting of the orthopedic clinic where anxiety, though present, was muted by routine procedures, social isolation was higher. In arthritis, where the long-range nature of the illness enabled family members to make active claims on clinic personnel, the sense of solidarity among family members was much higher.

It is interesting to compare these patterns with the rates of third person reference to physicians. In the orthopedic clinic, where references to physicians were frequent, first person plural usage by mothers was low. In the diabetic and especially in the cystic fibrosis clinics, where authority references to physicians were relatively infrequent, there was constant use of collective forms of expression. Arthritis represented an intermediate case where reference to physicians was fairly frequent but first person plural pronoun usage was also high.

This analysis suggests that as the authority of the physician increased, the relative strength of the family as a social unit declined. Conversely, as the sense of family solidarity was stronger, the reliance

[26] These variations in reliance on physicians' authority suggest only qualified support for Taylor's observation that nurses are expected to ride herd on doctors' implicit directives. Cf. C. Taylor, *In Horizontal Orbit: Hospitals and the Cult of Efficiency*, New York: Holt, Rinehart and Winston, 1970, *viz.* 115 ff.

[27] Cf. Appendix B, Table XV, Col. 6.

on the physician declined. In the orthopedic clinic, health authority was strongly vested in the physician. The power of the family to control the setting was at a minimum and the sense of social isolation was at its peak. At the opposite extreme was the cystic fibrosis clinic where the authority of the physician was weakest and the solidarity of the family was the most prominent.

VI-11. Effects of Children with Scoleosis Conditions

The presence of a certain number of families with children suffering from scoleosis reduced the bureaucratic character of the clinic, and made it necessary for nurses and physicians to take a more personal interest in families. These families often had to deal with serious surgery in the form of spinal fusion, along with the possibility of lifelong impairment to the children's posture. Nursing staff and physicians were familiar with these families, and spent considerable time with them in preparation for what to expect in the course of hospitalization, surgery and subsequent treatment. The nurse, in particular, spent longer periods alone with family members assuring them of her personal attention to the child while in the hospital. She also attempted to give emotional support, while giving a realistic assessment of the degree of correctability and the likely life-cycle consequences of the condition. She established a personal rapport which contrasted with the routine and rushed approach that was adopted with children suffering from ordinary orthopedic problems.

Children with scoleosis difficulties involved the nurse closely in the grave health care problems of these families. Intimate, supportive contacts with scoleosis families reduced the routine character of the clinic and provided an intense health care role for the nurse. Buttressed with this primary nursing function, she could assume the routine burdens in the clinic without loss of professional identity.

The presence of scoleosis families reduced the withdrawn and mechanical atmosphere of the clinic by enhancing the health care status of the nurse in the estimation of families. From this position as a helping person it was possible for the nurse, as a staff member with considerable seniority but with relatively little formal authority, to assume informal leadership. The focus of this leadership was in the administrative integration of the clinic.

VI-12. Medical Scope and Administrative Leadership Role

The scope of problems dealt with in the orthopedic clinic tended in a medical direction, although this trend was not as extreme as in the diabetic and cystic fibrosis services.[28] However, the rate of 67% treat-

[28] Cf. Appendix B, Table Ia, for percentages regarding scope of issues dealt with throughout the outpatient department.

ment of medical issues indicated a pattern consistent with a ritual structure of interaction.

The strong administrative leadership role played by the staff nurse was associated with the medical scope of problems. Many of the medical problems also had administrative dimensions. The self-assigned title of "traffic cop" fell to the nurse as a result of her constant battle for services. Her continuous struggle with the X-ray service and with the records room for information was posed at the level of medical scope, but was administrative in function. The orthopedic nurse by reason of long experience and familiarity with the hospital was well equipped for the task of wringing services for families from the various medical departments. Although these efforts were not always successful, families felt they had a resourceful advocate in the nurse.[29]

VI-13. Administrative Leadership and Bureaucratic Integration

In the highly bureaucratic and impersonal setting of the orthopedic clinic these nursing administrative services were of great importance. The weightiness of administration in the clinic is attested by the fact that the intensity of administrative activity conducted in the presence of families was higher than that in any other outpatient service.[30] Intensive administrative services were delivered to families in virtually every location within the hospital. These areas included the appointment desk, corridors, examination rooms, cast room, physician's offices and patient wards of the hospital. In no other clinic was administration carried directly to families on such a hospital-wide basis.

The value of this administrative service was not appreciated professionally by the nursing staff. Indeed, it was frequently asserted by the staff that with the move to the new building these administrative functions would be delegated to clerical personnel so that nurses would have more time to spend with families.

The data from the orthopedic clinic suggests a different appraisal of the nursing function there. In a large bureaucratic setting with many families clamoring for limited services, administration of necessity became a prime nursing function. In such a large scale service only through administrative leadership of a health identified person could the integration of care and cure functions be achieved. One of the principal care needs of families in the orthopedic clinic was help in con-

[29] The advocacy and mediation of the nurse served to reduce the dysfunctions of hierarchy as specified by Hall. Thus the mediation reduced both the inhibition of communication, and the necessity for approval of superordinates while it fostered the correction of errors. Cf. R. H. Hall, *Organizations: Structure and Process*, Englewood Cliffs, N. J.: Prentice-Hall, 1972.

[30] Cf. Appendix B, Table XVIII, for means for staff initiated administrative activity in the various clinics.

fronting the hospital bureaucracy. Only a senior nursing person, who had informal status but no formal authority, could be approached by families in the hope of getting a hearing for their pleas for hospital services. The administrative leadership of the nurse, even though not always successful in satisfying concrete family demands, achieved in some degree the functional integration of the cure and care systems of the clinic.[31]

VI-14. Affective Reservoir and Administrative Leadership

Patterns specific to the orthopedic clinic emerged in affective behavior by staff and families. These patterns were evidenced by intense levels of affective reserve accompanied by low degrees of affective expression. Affective behavior emerged in the absence of overt task activity, but feelings were not often expressed while definite action toward goals was in progress.[32] Courtship was relatively low during feedback opportunity and service, and small talk was most frequently in evidence in the absence of courtship. [33] The overall interactive pattern in the clinic was one of "affective isolation," with emotional behavior sharply separated from task activities.[34]

This pattern of affective isolation contrasted with that of restraint that characterized the arthritis clinic during the first year. Thus, in arthritis shown in Graph N-VI-14, though feelings were held in check overall, they tended to rise during work activities. This pattern was reversed during orthopedic interaction.

[31] The functional integration of the clinic was achieved through attempts to satisfy family demands from the inadequate supply of care. This suggested, for nursing, the role of "political broker." In accord with March's model the orthopedic nurse "negotiated" a position as "executive" leader in the clinic by paying "the price required for participation in the (political) coalition." Where administrative demands of staff and families were high, nursing "bargained" favorably in achieving "executive" leadership in the clinic "coalition". Cf. James G. March, "The Business Firm as a Political Coalition," *Journal of Politics,* XXIV (August, 1962), pp. 662-678.

[32] Indicated by a reservoir ratio of 1.081 and an expression ratio of 0.456. Cf. Appendix B, Table VII, Cols. 3 and 4.

[33] A reservoir ratio of 3.188 compared with an expression ratio of 0.938 suggested the isolation of courtship and small talk. Cf. Appendix B, Table IX, Cols. 4 and 5.

[34] This pattern of "affective isolation" was particularly prominent in the examination rooms where joking behavior was frequently reserved for the termination of interviews. It closely resembles the ecological control of expression of pain described by Rosengren and De Vault, "The Sociology of Time and Space in an Obstetrical Hospital," in Freidson, *The Hospital in Modern Society,* especially p. 284.

The tendency for feelings to be expressed in isolation from orthopedic task activities was related at once to the underlying tensions in the system and to the administrative integration accomplished by nursing leadership. Personnel shortages, cramped quarters and inadequate medical leadership were institutional tension-building factors. These institutional strains served to aggravate the underlying anxieties of families confronting orthopedic problems. The necessity for the head nurse to confront and placate irate parents represented a

GRAPH N-VI-14

Components of Affective Behavior in the Orthopedic and Arthritis Clinics during the First Year

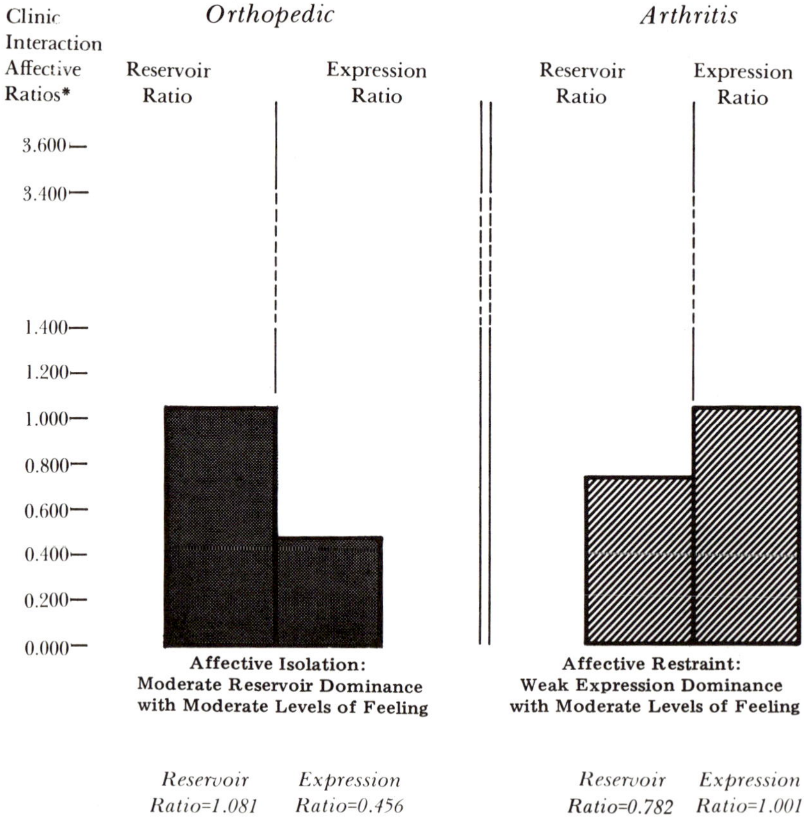

**Based on ratios presented in Table VII, Appendix B, p. 207.*

conjunction of these organizational and family difficulties. The use of small talk, apart from task performance, performed a tension release role. Both for families and for staff these emotional expressions had a value in reducing conflicts.[35]

VI-15. Humor and Ritual Patterns of Affective Behavior

The occurrence of small talk in isolation from task activities was coupled with the frequent use of humor. Sometimes humor was used to establish social distance and to avoid involvement with complex, emotional problems. Humor, however, was frequently used to break log jams and to adjudicate disputes. On such occasions no direct practical result might take place, but humor was employed to establish greater tolerance of conflict situations.

Humor was also often used as an expression of ritualized attitudes. The self-assigned designation of the nurse as "traffic cop" had this ritualized effect. The title because of its demeaning and self-deprecating appearance, served to establish beliefs about the authoritarian character of the clinic. Given the bureaucratic and confused state of the service, the need for exercise of arbitrary police power was evident. The deprecatory title served to establish the nurse's exercise of power and to make it acceptable.

Humor was also used in a bantering manner with children as a ritualized form of soliciting their courage in putting up with orthopedic problems. These humorous exchanges also were ritualized expressions of the nurse's need for strength in dealing with children's problems.

The isolation of humor from work activities emphasized its ritual nature. It was used in a symbolic manner to express institutional attitudes. These attitudes included the desire of the staff to maintain social distance, and to establish order in a large bureaucratic service. The emphasis on courage highlighted authority and signalled the avoidance of intimacy. The use of humor to express these institutional attitudes implied an individualistic value approach. Each family was expected to accept these attitudes individually. The use of humor as a means of communicating institutional assumptions was an individualized ritual procedure.

VI-16. Ritual Control and Unstructured Roles

The ritualized use of humor for attitude communication was accompanied by a moderately low level of interactive role assignment. De-

[35] This management of strains in administrative leadership is suggestive of system tensions, which are regarded by Buckley as endemic and energizing to adaptive systems. Cf. Buckley, *Sociology and Modern Systems Theory*, p. 51.

spite the large size of the clinic, differentiation of roles was less articulated in orthopedics than in the smaller arthritis clinic during the first period of the research.[36] The lesser amount of role structuring in orthopedic interaction as compared with arthritis is shown in Graph O-VI-16. A factor in this reduced structuring was the dominance of small talk by the staff during activities with orthopedic families. In arthritis, on the other hand, families assumed the usual outpatient role by initiating more intensive levels of small talk than did the staff. The relative absence of role structuring was traceable to the frequent absence of prior contact between orthopedic staff and families. Families assumed various interactive attitudes according to situational requirements with staff control reduced through lack of prior design.

The general absence of fixed interactive structuring was connected with the affective patterns that have been discussed. The isolated use of small talk was related to the management of strain arising from adventitious role patterning. The ritualized use of humor as a device for attitude communication seemed suited to deal with anomic, ill-defined situations. The need for ritual humor in the service of administrative leadership was reinforced by the existence of a fluid interactive structure.

VI-17. Ritual, Family Initiative and Home Issues

As indicated in the qualitative discussion of family interviews, there was a strong tendency for families to introduce home-related issues, and for staff to focus on medical or hospital problems. During examination room contacts families were responsible for 50.5% of home scope discussion, but only 34.0% of medical issues. The tendency of families to discuss home problems was found throughout the outpatient services.[37]

In the orthopedic clinic this conflict between staff and family concerns was dealt with through ritualized affective patterns. Strains arising from family fears and social stresses were handled through the ritualized isolation of feelings. Small talk was expressed independently of courtship, and the latter tended to occur separately from feedback processes and service activities. Conflict between family interests and hospital interests was handled through ritual humor. Families were told in ritual form that home problems were not the concern of the hospital ("not that much my business").

[36] As shown by an overall staff-family correlation difference in the four feedback-related variables of 0.911, as compared with a total difference of 1.296 in arthritis. Cf. Appendix B, Table IV, for lagged correlations from the orthopedic and arthritis clinics.

[37] Cf. Appendix B, Table II.

GRAPH O-VI-16

Role Structuring in the Orthopedic and Arthritis Clinics during the First Year

(medical scope interaction*)

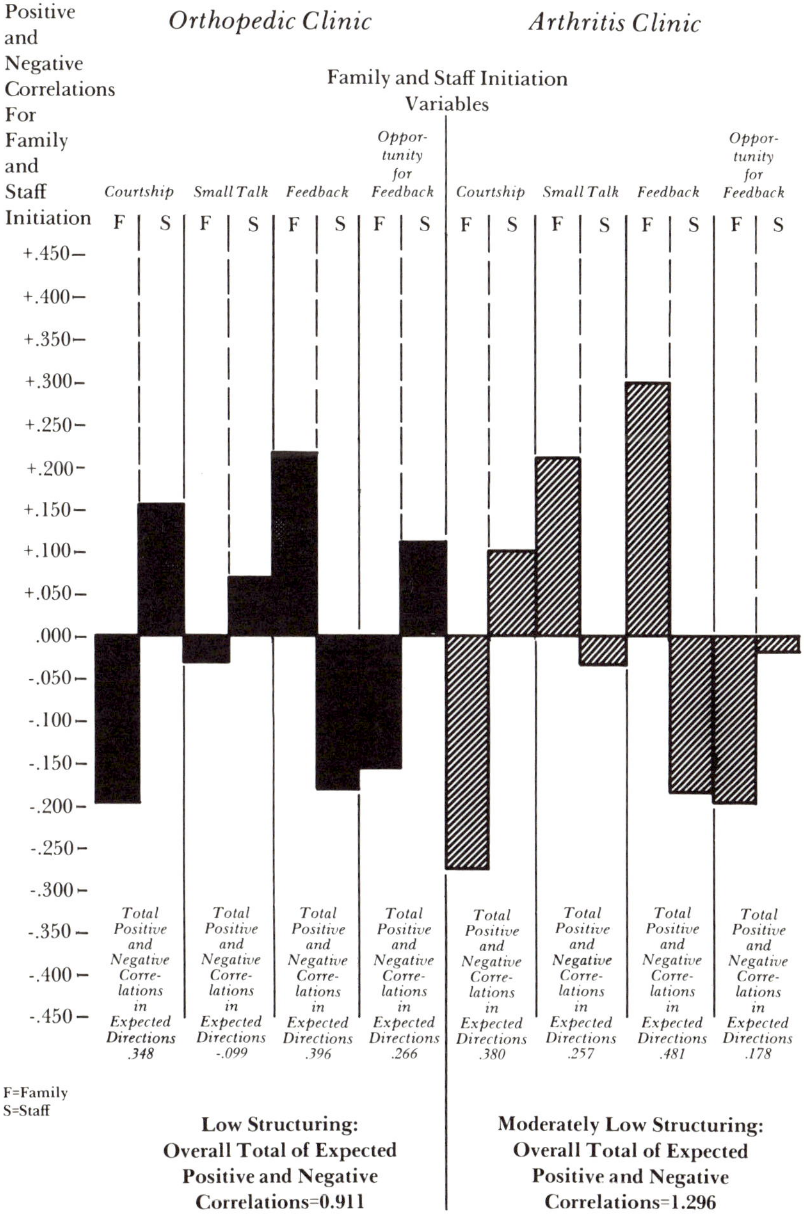

**Based on lagged correlations as presented in Table V, Appendix B, p. 206.*

The ritualized use of humor in fending off family initiated discussion of home problems fell to the lot of the nurse as an extension of her administrative role. The use of humor in this capacity was an effort to soften the institutional blow to family feelings. The fact that there were really organizational constraints forcing the staff to rush family treatment, partly justified this behavior. At times, however, ritualized responses to home-related and personal issues seemed examples of bureaucratic and medical defensiveness.[38]

VI-18. Improvising Elements in a Ritual Response Structure

The interactive network of the orthopedic clinic displayed improvising elements in a ritual response system. A relatively undifferentiated interactive structure characterized staff-family conferences. Home and life cycle problems constituted 33% of the content of interaction, a level considerably higher than that in diabetes (13%) and cystic fibrosis (11%) during the first year. Also overall family initiative provided 36.7% of interaction, a figure exceeded only by that of the arthritis service (44.3%).[39]

Despite these improvising elements, interaction took place within the institutional bonds of a system defined by ritualized affect.The isolation of feelings from work related activities weakened family initiative and inhibited home-issue discussion. The ritualized use of humor maintained social distance and institutionalized norms of authority and laconic acceptance of orthopedic problems. Humor itself institutionalized the norm of individual acceptance of clinic attitudes.

VI-19. Ritualized Affect, Administrative Integration and Feedback Response

The use of ritualized, reserved affect played an important role in the administrative area and in the communication process with families. The nurse's function as "traffic cop" and adjudicator of disputes between staff and families was energized by ritualized types of forensic humor. Breaking administrative log-jams called for public forms of humor with the nurse as judge and jury. Draconian impulses were rationalized by the need to "keep the clinic running smoothly."

Ritualized forms of reserved affect also played an important part in the direction of health services delivered to families. Ritualized affect, indicated by isolation of small talk and courtship from task activities, served to reduce strains in staff-family contacts caused by organiza-

[38] Cf. I. Menzies, "A Case Study in the Functioning of Social Systems as a Defense Against Anxiety: A report on a study of the nursing service," *Human Relations,* XIII (May, 1960), pp. 95-121.

[39] Cf. Appendix B, Table II.

tional constraints. These constraints included limitations on staff time and staff need to emphasize medical rather than home-related problems. The conflict and tension between staff and families over the need to discuss medical rather than social and emotional issues was reduced by ritualized small talk and humor. The function of the ritual was to underline the need of the staff to focus on medical problems and to induce family acceptance of this limitation. The public role of the nurse as administrative integrator and judge provided support for the private ritual role in inducing this acceptance. The private role in family communication was a normative extension of the public role as a symbol of the institutional norms of the orthopedic clinic.

The effectiveness of the private ritualized role of the nurse was evidenced by the patterns of feedback process. When analysis was made of feedback a rather high degree of feedback sensitivity was observed.[40] Moreover, staff and families shared equally in this high sensitivity to requests for information.[41]

When a first year comparison is made with arthritis the feedback responsiveness was higher in the orthopedic clinic, as shown in Graph P-VI-19. Thus higher overall and average family and staff response occurred in orthopedics. Moreover a virtually even balance of orthopedic responsiveness contrasted with a heavy staff dominance in arthritis.

The ritualized affective role of the nurse played a significant part in this pattern of feedback response. Through ritual use of small talk and humor the nurse focused communication on medical problems with which the staff was prepared to deal. Through ritual affective tactics, interest in home and life-cycle issues was dampened, and conflict from these issues was muted. With attention ritually focused on medical problems, communication with families could proceed effectively, as indicated by the rather high level of mutual feedback response attained.[42]

VI-20. Alternative Coping Procedures

The use of affective ritual to focus on medical problems was partly a means of denying long-term anxieties of parents relating to life time

[40] Indicated by an average family-staff feedback response of 25.2% (as measured by unique variances from the lagged regression analysis). Cf. Appendix B, Table VI.

[41] *Ibid.*

[42] Mutual feedback patterns between staff and families, suggest that despite muted feelings, persuasion and care functions as specified by Freidson were present. Cf. E. Freidson, *Professional Dominance: The Social Structure of Medical Care,* N. Y.: Atherton Press, 1970, p. 120.

body damage to their children. In most cases these fears were unfounded physically. The staff tried to diminish them by instilling confidence in orthopedic medicine. Insofar as exaggerated fears were warded off, reality controlled communication (as indicated by the sensitivity of feedback processes). Through reality control of the feedback process (in the context of organic and institutional limitations) the clinic was effective in helping families cope with life issues. The ability to distinguish real from unreal life time problems is characteristic of coping systems.

This ability was manifested by the higher level of feedback responsiveness that was a feature of communication with scoleosis families. Interviews with these families attained the highest level of feedback response observed in the outpatient department.[43] The greater sensitiv-

[43] This was shown by an average family-staff feedback response of 31.0%. Cf. Appendix B, Table VI.

GRAPH P-VI-19

Feedback Responsiveness by Families and Staff in the Orthopedic and Arthritis Clinics during the First Year

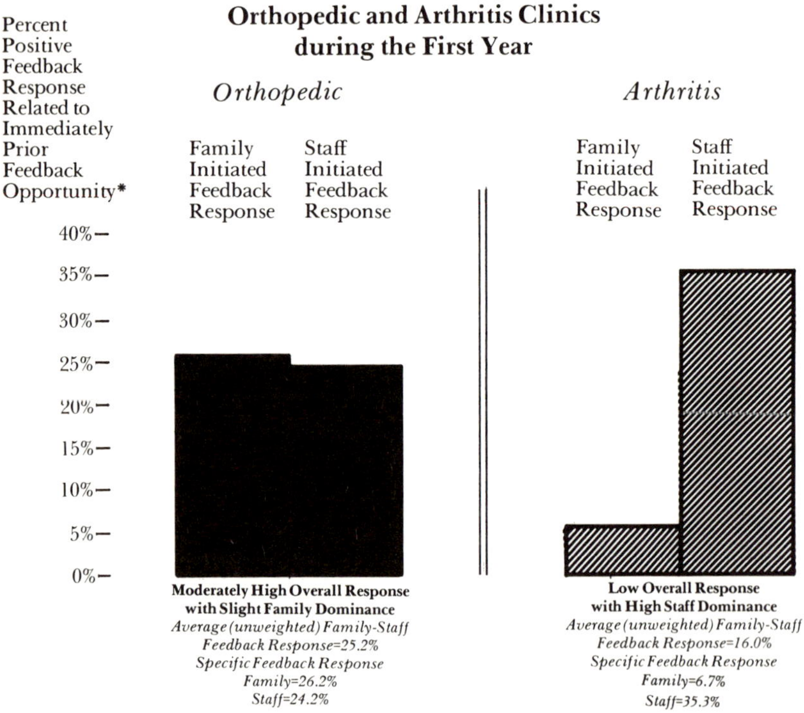

**Based on lagged regression analysis of data presented in Table VI, Appendix B, p. 207.*

ity of communication and the greater attention given to these families indicated the ability of the clinic to discriminate between real and unreal bases for lifetime fears. The use of ritualized humor expressed symbolically the capacity of the clinic to make this reality judgment. The general absence of humor during interviews with scoleosis families indicated the ability of the clinic to cope by alternative means with life-cycle issues. With scoleosis families ritualized denial of lifetime injury was replaced by greater openness in intensified mutual feedback on life-cycle consequences of the children's condition.

VI-21. Flexible Coping Mechanisms and Effective Support

The ability to develop alternate means of assisting families in coping with varied life-cycle issues marked the clinic as an effective support setting. The use of humor, along with discussion focused on the short-term nature of routine orthopedic problems, did serve to reduce family fears of possible long-term consequences of the child's condition. At the same time, the open mutual feedback process between staff and families, given clinic time constraints, was evidence of two-way communication. The focus of this communication was family fears of long-term injury to the child. Mutual feedback response tended to allay these anxieties through staff assurances of the effectiveness and short-term nature of the medical treatment. Although there were cases of avoidance of reality-based long-term fears, such instances were exceptional. Most cases were short-term in nature, and the sensitive use of humor and open feedback communication appeared to provide effective support for families' need to rely on an effective medical technology.

The ability of the staff to adopt a long-term life cycle approach with scoleosis families indicated the flexibility of the clinic as a coping setting. Parents and children were carefully and sensitively instructed in the degree of correction that might be expected from a spinal fusion operation. Examples of other children who had completed this ordeal were discussed. The process of hospitalization, before and after the operation, was gone into thoroughly, with frequent questions from parent and child marking the discussions. Encouragement was provided in the form of realistic assessment of the period of hospitalization and after-care treatment. The personal commitment of the nurse to the child during the hospitalization, and operative and post-operative care, was warmly and personally expressed. The absence of humor and intensified mutual feedback between family and nurse provided empirical evidence of the support provided to these families coping with long-term scoleosis problems.

VI-22. The Orthopedic Clinic: A Staff Based Ritual Organization

Insofar as the orthopedic clinic was able to develop alternative mechanisms for dealing with fears based on real and unreal threats of life-time bodily injury, it was a coping sub-system. Since most problems in the clinic were short run in nature, the prevalence of ritualized affect characterized the overall functioning of the clinic.

From the staff perspective the choice of the examination room as location for health care was in the interest of individualized care sought by families themselves. From the perspective of coping systems, the staff base limited response to medical problems and avoided unreal fears of life-time problems. (At times the staff base was overused to deny life-time problems which were founded in reality.) The effectiveness of ritualized small talk and humor in overcoming these fears may be seen in the sensitive feedback process in the clinic. The decline of humor and ritualized affect, accompanied by increased feedback responsiveness during interaction with scoleosis families indicated the capacity of the clinic to provide flexible support for different life-cycle issues.

CHAPTER VII

THE ORTHOPEDIC CLINIC: CHANGE IN A STAFF BASED RITUAL ORGANIZATION

Important changes were introduced into the orthopedic clinic with the move to the new site. The facilities were far better suited to the technical needs of families. In place of three examination rooms, ten were now available. There were also testing and laboratory facilities, offices for physicians, a nursing station, a conference room and a residents' room for the convenience of the clinic staff. A wide pair of hallways connected by an intersecting passage gave an H-form to the medical areas providing ready access to the various parts of the clinic. At the entrance to the parallel hallways stood a large administration desk with files and computer information on visiting families. Facing the administration desk, reached by elevator from the ground floor, a large waiting room with comfortable couches and chairs had been attractively arranged, with blackboards and small tables for children to use while waiting for their appointments. (See Figure C-III-1, p. 34, above.)

The staff of the clinic had been augmented by the addition of several more physicians, a nursing assistant, a second administrative clerk and a part-time recreational assistant who helped waiting families take care of their children. A clinic administrator was now in charge of supplies and performed many of the administrative tasks formerly managed by the head nurse.

As explained by the nurse, who continued in her capacity as senior person responsible for orthopedic nursing services, an average of about forty families were seen each day, in morning and afternoon sessions. The general practice was to schedule appointments for approximately sixty families between 10 a.m. and 5 p.m., five days a week. Of those scheduled, approximately one third usually failed to appear, but, the nurse explained, "sometimes most of them show up . . . last Friday, 62 came in between 11 a.m. and 6 p.m." The staff nurse commented ruefully to the observer that "we do get hit like that occasionally. I don't know who accomplishes what on a day like that!"

The additional staff in the new clinic diminished the involvement of the head nurse in administrative activities. In characterizing the new clinic she said to the observer: "It [is] kind of . . . patient-oriented, to a degree, but in the old clinic I used to have to fight with the record man or the x-ray department to get them . . . and I just can't do that any more . . . I try to stay away from this mess as much as possible except to go through the charts to see who is coming up."

With the availability of new technical installations the head nurse received computer print-outs about children scheduled for each current clinic session, indicating, for example, whether they needed x-rays, whether they were to see a particular physician, or whether the visiting nurses association had made some inquiry about them.

It was expected that routine administrative duties would be taken over by the new clerical staff. Thus, the intensity of administrative activities had decreased rather sharply.[1]

VII-1. Change in Length and Amount of Family Contact

Despite the diminished involvement in administration, a decline occurred in the overall amount of nursing time devoted to family contact in the new orthopedic clinic. A decrease from 43.6% to 41.7% in time given to interaction with families took place, although the number of families contacted increased from 90 in the first year to 116 in the second. The average length of family interviews was reduced from 11.8 minutes to 7.3 minutes in the new clinic.

Although a few conferences lasted over half an hour, there was a trend toward brief meetings lasting only for a couple of minutes. Many of these encounters were purely social.[2] These brief contacts tended to avoid complex social issues, suggesting that a pattern of defensiveness had emerged in the new clinic.

[1] As shown by a decline from a staff mean initiation of 1.189, to 1.028 in the new orthopedic clinic. Cf. Appendix B, Table XVIII.

[2] The greatest amount of social behavior (25.3%) was recorded in the orthopedic clinic during the second year. Cf. Appendix B, Table XVII, showing that percentages of social activities in the other services were, 5.4% in cystic fibrosis, 5.1% in arthritis, and 4.4% in diabetes.

VII-2. Changes in Staff-Family Location Usage

Along with the decline in overall family contact, and the contraction in the duration of family conferences, there were decided shifts in the use of various locations for both staff-family and intra-staff activities.

Areas of staff-family and intra-staff interaction are front, back or interstitial regions.[3] The front region in which families were usually contacted, and in which staff engaged in prepared conferences with parents and children constituted the examination rooms of the orthopedic clinic.[4] These areas contrasted with back locations such as the physicians' offices, residents' room, nursing station and staff conference rooms, where family members were never present. Interstitial to these front and back orthopedic areas were the waiting room, administration desk, corridors, cast room and in-patient wards of the hospital. Here casual meetings might occur between staff and families.[5]

As in the first year, the examination rooms were marked by the highest frequency of family contact. In fact the amount of staff-family activity increased slightly in the cure center of the clinic from 83% in the first, to 89% in the second year.[6]

VII-3. Changes in Staff Location Use

Activities between staff members not involving families took place in both front and back areas of the hospital. Contacts involving only staff declined from 32.3% to 22.8% in interstitial areas where families had access. On the other hand such intra-staff meetings in the back areas increased with the move to the new clinic from 24.1% to 35.5%. The trend was for staff to meet more frequently where no families were ever found, and less often where families might be encountered.[7]

[3] Cf. Goffman, *Presentation of Self in Everyday Life*. Cf. also *Asylums* and *Encounters: Two Studies in the Sociology of Interaction,* Indianapolis: Bobbs Merrill, 1961.

[4] Cf. W. R. Rosengren and S. De Vault, "The Sociology of Time and Space in an Obstetrical Hospital," in Freidson, *The Hospital in Modern Society,* especially pp. 276-285, for use of specialized medical areas by staff to maintain "tempo, timing and rhythm".

[5] Cf. Rosengren and De Vault, *op. cit.,* p. 289, for discussion of the importance of interstitial areas as locations of "casual contact," where "performance" management is less salient.

[6] Cf. Appendix B, Table Ib.

[7] This avoidance of interstitial areas for interstaff encounters is in accord with Mechanic's suggestion that rules are used by lower participants as "chips" in a bargaining process. The avoidance of the waiting room, administration desk and corridors was an implicit adherence to the rule that nursing was not to be involved in the "mess" of negotiations between families and hospital services. Cf. Mechanic, "Sources of Power of Lower Participants in Complex Organizations," *Administrative Science Quarterly,* VII (December, 1962) p. 349.

VII-4. Changes in Interstitial Area Family Contact

Interstitial areas, such as the waiting room, appointment desk, corridors, cast room and in-patient wards of the hospital were locations where chance contacts occurred with families.[8] Here families frequently used the opportunity for casual meetings to raise problems of an administrative nature which they encountered in obtaining services from the hospital. Use of these areas as places of contact between staff and families fell from 12% during the first period to 5% in the second.[9] Along with a decline in the number of these unscheduled meetings, there was also a reduction in the intensity of administrative activities in these areas.[10] This trend was in line with the observation of the nurse that responsibility for the "mess" of administrative problems had largely been passed on to clerical personnel.

Increased nursing back area activity had a trend toward greater involvement with staff other than physicians. With the relinquishing of an important role in the administrative control of the clinic, nursing contact with clerical, supervisory and social service personnel moved away from interstitial areas of casual contact with families.[11] In these back area conferences the orthopedic nurse exercised some political influence over subordinate members of the hospital staff.[12] Interpersonal sway over minor personnel within the hospital bureaucracy replaced the administrative leadership role assumed by nursing during the prior year.[13]

VII-5. Trends in Cure Center Family Contact

The removal of the burden of administration carried on in the interstitial areas of the hospital, freed the nursing staff for steady contact with families in the examination rooms. Several such family meetings suggest, however, that the quality of health services was not greatly

[8] Cf. Footnote 5 above.

[9] Cf. Appendix B, Table Ib.

[10] Thus the mean for administrative interaction with families in these interstitial areas declined in the new clinic (from 1.453 to 1.151).

[11] Cf. Rosengren and De Vault, "The Sociology of Time and Space in an Obstetrical Hospital," *op. cit.*, p. 289.

[12] In accordance with Goffman's analysis, impressions fostered by performances with families in the examination room were "knowingly contradicted" in these back areas by the staff "as a matter of course." Cf. Goffman, *The Presentation of Self in Everyday Life,* p. 106. Greater status for staff is attributed to back areas by Rosengren and De Vault, *op. cit.*, p. 279.

[13] Thompson specifies a variety of conditions under which discretionary personnel tend not to take new initiatives. Cf. J. D. Thompson, *Organizations in Action,* pp. 127 ff.

changed from that observed during the first year. Among the shortcomings in the previous period were the inability to identify or deal with socially related problems of significant physical consequence to children's health, and the failure to make appropriate referrals of problems to social service or to community health resources. Due to continued failure to plan for family conferences by use of clinic notes or staff consultation, similar deficiencies were evident during staff-family meetings in the new clinic.

An example of these difficulties is presented by a mother and her eight-year-old son, who attended the clinic accompanied by a physical therapist from their home community. The relationship between the family and the physical therapist is evident as is the staff's attitude toward clinic health care:

Nurse to physical therapist: And you don't need any new orders now, do you?

Physical therapist to nurse: No, except you had sent me a copy last time [last words inaudible].

Doctor to physical therapist: Let's see, as long as we see him [blank] about every six weeks, I suppose.

Nurse to herself: Now that'll be . . .

[**Transcriber's comment:** Doctor says something inaudible.]

Nurse to doctor: O.K. Thank you.

Doctor to nurse: O.K.?

[**Transcriber's comment:** The door is opened and closed after the doctor leaves.]

Physical therapist to nurse: The doctor didn't mention it, but can he go back to school, right away, do you think?

Nurse to physical therapist: He should go to school. Ah huh, and with his pillow. Do you have anything to do with the school nurse out there?

Physical therapist to nurse: I don't know her. [Last words inaudible, something about usually contacting the school.]

Nurse to physical therapist: Uh, huh, is there usually any contact between you?

Physical therapist to nurse: I usually get in contact with them, in contact with the school. Mostly they call me up at the apartment. [Short laugh.]

Nurse to physical therapist: Right. So I can either write another referral for them, which is essentially the same as the one to you, or if the nurse that follows them wants to convey it,—

Physical therapist to nurse: It doesn't make any difference. Yes. Uh huh.

Nurse to physical therapist: There always should be a call to the school nurse regarding the orders.

Physical therapist to nurse: I think I could let Miss James handle that, I think they know her best.

Nurse to physical therapist: Fine.

Physical therapist to nurse: So we could start today and [several words inaudible]. I don't think that would be a problem.

Nurse to physical therapist: Even on the playground he's not limited, except to contact sports which they don't usually have at this age. But he's as good as the next guy really. And if he falls he's not going to fall any more than the next guy, I'm sure. They become very versatile in it. [She laughs.]

[**Transcriber's comment:** The physical therapist says something inaudible.]

Nurse to physical therapist: It wouldn't be fair to make him sit in the classroom while the other kids were out there.

Physical therapist to nurse: O.K. All right.

It is evident that neither physician nor nurse made any effort to enlist the interest or responsibility of the mother in the care of this young boy. Neither during nor after the contact with the family did the staff try to speak to the physical therapist about the possibility of further involving the mother. The staff assumed that the therapist had taken charge of the care of the child. No effort was made to anticipate what might occur if the services of the therapist or of community health personnel were to be interrupted. The possible social consequences of this dependency pattern, though identified by the nurse to the observer, were thought of as outside the competence of the clinic.

VII-6. An Example of Avoidance of Home Related Issues

A further example of the neglect of home-related problems was presented by a conversation of the nurse with a mother who was accompanied by her five-month-old son. The child, in addition to his orthopedic problem, was suffering from cerebral palsy. To enable the mother to bring the child to the clinic, the father had to arrange to come home from work early to take care of the three other pre-school boys. The nurse questioned the mother about arrangements for bringing all the children in for various immunization shots, and suggested the possibility of a morning appointment. To this proposal the mother responded as follows:

Mother to nurse: It's impossible in the mornings. The only time I can go in is in the afternoons.

Nurse to mother: Well [in a questioning tone]...

Mother to nurse: Well, I know I can make . . . I know [pause]

Nurse to mother: Well, you've got your choice.

Mother to nurse: Ah . . . I'm going to make an appointment, actually, for tomorrow, 'cos I know my husband will be home tomorrow. He has more worries, actually when they come down here because he has to . . . has to take time off from work.

Nurse to mother: Um hm.

Mother to nurse *(continuing):* To come home, see? I mean, come down here, he had to come home to mind the other kids and either come down here. So, he'll be home . . . he'll be home about four-thirty tomorrow. He's planning on going to the [ticket office] over in Oakville.

Nurse to mother: Oh. You've got more problems than I'd like to have. I'll tell you that!

[Both nurse and mother laugh in a friendly fashion.]

Mother to nurse: Well, he buys a ticket and he wants to go, so . . .

Nurse to mother: Uh ha. Yea.

Mother to nurse: He'll go there, but . . . I don't know, anyway.

Nurse to mother: Well, You see what you can do. You've got your choice. You've got your private [doctor]. You can always go down to Ridge Avenue.

Mother to nurse *(interrupting):* Oh! I know. Oh, yes, I know that! But I have . . . I . . . as I say . . . I . . . I will get over!

Nurse to mother: But, if you . . . yes . . . it's like . . . a . . . it's like the old saying that . . .

Mother to nurse: I know!

Nurse to mother *(continuing):* People who say they're not going to get married until they can afford to and so they never do![14]

[14] This comment in the context of the problems of this family in keeping clinic appointments had the effect of isolating the husband. In the context of strain on nurse and mother, this suggests an involuntary adoption of Bond and

Mother to nurse: Uh ha. That's true. [Laughs nervously.]

Nurse to mother: And this is the same thing. If you don't get the shots until you have the time to do so, you never will.

Mother to nurse: Well, I . . . I have the time, if I could only get . . . if I could only get in!

Nurse to mother: You've got a lot of little ones. That's it.

Mother to nurse: No. If I could only get out of the door . . . If I got a lot of . . . what you say . . . and . . .

Nurse to mother: And you have to go back for more shots, too.

Mother to nurse: Even today.

Nurse to mother: Sure!

Mother to nurse *(continuing her sentence):* I[t] was a hard time getting down here, believe me!

Nurse to mother: Yea. I noticed you missed the last one.

Mother to nurse *(interrupting):* The last one I missed. And I didn't even know I had . . .

Mother to nurse: . . . couldn't even have thought of it! To tell you the truth, I forgot all about it! [Pause.] You know, the better kids can watch . . . I just forget. I just [her voice trails off]—the appointment. He has been cutting teeth and he's been so crabby!

Nurse to mother: You're busy just changing pants!

The nursing approach to this family was similar to that in the previous year in its avoidance of social and emotional problems.

The striking degree of tension that developed between mother and nurse, was communicated to the child, who started to cry vociferously. The stress derived in part from the narrow focus on medical aspects of the situation as indicated by the nurse's concern with immunization shots. The level of tension increased as the interview progressed, the conference covering about thirty minutes. In the first year, when the nurse was constantly involved in administrative activities, a detached attitude toward the situation could more readily be maintained by escape from the interaction when strains began to mount.

Vinacke's observation that "two weak (female) members tend to ally against the stronger when this strategy can win." Since the father was absent his "stronger" position was weakened which made him a ready target for scapegoating brought on by the anxiety of the nurse. Cf. John R. Bond and W. Edgar Vinacke, "Coalitions in Mixed Sex Triads," *Sociometry,* XXIV (March, 1961), pp. 61-75.

In the new clinic, such escape was not readily available. The nurse referred to the physician as a means of relieving the situation, but when the mother continued to look for assistance, the nurse responded with a vague effort at social support. However, at no time did she attempt to relieve the family's distress by suggestions, for instance, about transportation. This failure, along with the failure to suggest other helping services, is traced to the fact that no planning of interviews was made based on study of clinic notes or on staff consultation.

This interaction suggests the concern of families with home related problems and the tendency for staff to place emphasis on medical scope issues. This was typical of such examination room contacts as shown by a continued family pattern of home scope initiation and staff initiation of medical issues. Thus, content of interactive patterning remained much unchanged from the previous year.[15]

VII-7. Interstitual Area Use and Affective Ritual

A tendency for meetings with families to take place in a structured manner in the clinic examination rooms, accompanied staff retreat to back areas. This trend was associated with a decline of administrative assistance to families in interstitial areas.[16]

Activities were divided between front and back areas where well-defined orthopedic activities took place.[17] The pattern indicated the

[15] Cf. Appendix B, Table II, showing 31.2% family medical initiation, and 51.3% family initiative at home scope during examination room interaction, as compared with figures of 34.0% and 50.5% for these types of family activities in the first year.

[16] As seen by Rosengren and De Vault interstitial areas appeared solely as regions of interstaff contact. These areas were places of casual meeting with no audiences when performances were neither enacted, nor "knowingly contradicted". In the orthopedic clinic contacts occurred in the corridors and at the administration desk between staff and families in "out-of-role" situations, where informal bargains were negotiated. This region of administrative turmoil had been the locus of nursing leadership in the old orthopedic clinic. Cf. Rosengren and De Vault, op. cit. p. 289. The concept of interstitial area is closely related to that of "interactional territories" defined as any place where a social gathering may occur. It was consequently a place where persons could meet in a manner outside their formally assigned social roles. Cf. Lyman and Scott, "Territoriality: A Neglected Sociological Dimension," *Sociology of the Absurd.*

[17] Goffman speaks of the importance of the separation of front and back regions. This assertion appears to be made more from the viewpoint of the staff than of families. From the standpoint of coping institutions, in which families are viewed as active members of the system, importance is assigned to interstitial areas where "performances" are minimized and roles are less sharpened during informal contact and negotiation. Cf. Goffman, *The Presentation of Self in Everyday Life,* p. 124.

avoidance of interstitial areas of casual contact between orthopedic families and staff, such as the waiting room, administration desk and corridors of the clinic.[18]

The interstitial regions of a large, bureaucratic clinic such as the orthopedic service are the integrative areas of the health system. Here the needs of families in seeking services intersect with the needs of the hospital as an institutional structure. The functional issue that is negotiated here is the allocation of scarce services among seekers and providers of these services.

The interstitial areas in the old orthopedic clinic were a zone of conflict (an area of "this mess" in the words of the head nurse). The effort to adjudicate disputes and to break administrative log-jams had defined the self-styled role of the nurse as "traffic cop." Associated with this authority role was a pattern of ritualized affect characterized by the large scale use of feelings, especially as indicated by small talk, for the release of tension.[19]

With the move of the clinic, the control over the interstitial area was largely surrendered to administrative assistants. With the reduction of administrative activities a parallel decrease was noted in ritualized affect.[20] The ritual patterns that occurred in the prior year showed that feelings were employed to relieve tension and to manage conflict and hostility but were not primarily used for work on concrete tasks. The abandonment of the integrative clinic areas coincided with the breakup of these ritual affective patterns, with overall feelings declining and affective reservoir falling sharply relative to expression.[21]

[18] Back stage is spoken of by Goffman as "free areas" where there is release from the usual routine. However, this freedom is closely circumscribed by the deliberate contradiction of front stage performances. This clearly marked staff role behavior contrasts with the casual informal behavior that occurs in interstitial areas where there is "no audience". Cf. Goffman, *Asylums,* pp. 227-237. Cf. also Rosengren and De Vault op. cit. p. 289 for discussion of interstitial areas as regions of casual contact for conflict resolution.

[19] Goffman speaks of the need for milieu therapy where status barriers are lowered. In the old orthopedic clinic interstitial areas appeared to have functioned in this therapeutic manner. Goffman, *The Presentation of Self in Everyday Life,* p. 199.

[20] Reserved feelings, indicated by small talk and courtship exerted in the absence of task activities, fell noticeably (indicated by a reservoir ratio decline from 1.081 to 0.379). A slight increase in the expression of feelings during work activities from 0.456 to 0.588 resulted in an overall decline of mean affect (from 0.769 to 0.486) with expressed exceeding reserved feelings (by 0.209).

[21] For a related discussion of use of medical areas and staff dominance of interaction as defenses against anxiety, Cf. I. Menzies, "A Case Study in the Functioning of Social Systems as a Defense against Anxiety: A report on a study of the nursing service," *Human Relations,* XIII (May, 1960), pp. 95-121.

The decline in overall feelings, and in particular the fall in affective reservoir, are shown in Graph Q-VII-7. These declines contrast with the rises in emotions that may be noted in arthritis. Thus whereas emotional restriction befell the orthopedic clinic, a freer and higher toned expression of affective channelling took place in arthritis.

GRAPH Q-VII-7

Change in Components of Affective Behavior in the Orthopedic and Arthritis Clinics

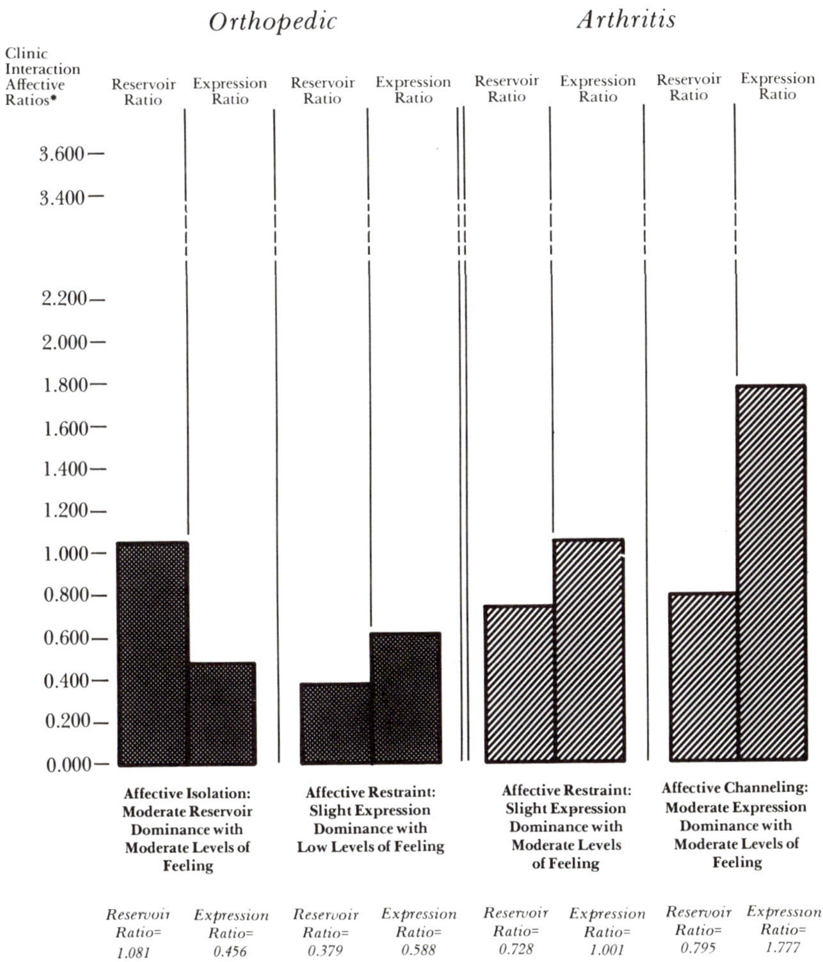

**Based on Ratios presented in Table VII, Appendix B, p. 207.*

VII-8. Medical Scope and Staff Control

With the move there developed a tendency for home-related problems to receive somewhat greater attention during family interviews. Medical issues declined in interactive concern (from 67% to 62%) while home and life-cycle problems increased in importance (from 33% to 38%).[22]

However, in examination room interaction no important change occurred in the tendency of families to dominate home-related problem discussion. In fact families were more active in initiating home and life cycle issues while staff increased slightly its activity relating to medical problems.[23] Differences centering on family concern with non-technical issues and staff preference for medical problems continued unabated. This maintenance of the level of content of staff and family concerns contrasted with the arthritis clinic. In arthritis definite increases were observed in family activity relating to medical topics, and in staff involvement in non-medical concerns.

Thus Graph R-VII-8 indicates that in arthritis medical scope interaction evolved from intense to slight staff control. In orthopedics, however, an initially strong control of such interaction became even more dominated by the staff.

VII-9. Decline in Feedback Responsiveness and De-Integration

The increased staff control of orthopedic family interaction suggested a more routinized ritual activity. This was related to the loss, with the move to the new clinic, of the integrative function provided by nursing administrative leadership.

More rigid interactive behavior and loss of institutional integration was associated with a significant decline in feedback responsiveness. While staff response to feedback opportunity increased slightly from 24.2% to 25.7%, family feedback response fell sharply from 26.2% to 9.1%. This was the sharpest decline in responsiveness shown in any of the clinics, and resulted in nearly the lowest average response (17.4%) during the course of the research.[24]

This decline in overall responsiveness, and especially the fall of family involvement in the feedback process, contrasts with the trends observed in arthritis as shown in Graph S-VII-9. The rise in arthritis family feedback response was related to increased affective channelling

[22] Cf. Appendix B, Table Ia.

[23] Shown by a slight family rise in home initiation from 50.5% to 51.3% and a life cycle increase from 38.8% to 43.1%. Family medical initiative declined from 34.0% to 31.2%. Cf. Appendix B, Table II, for examination room interaction analysis.

[24] Cf. Appendix B, Table VI.

GRAPH R-VII-8

Changes in Family and Staff Control of Scope of Examination Room Interaction in the Orthopedic and Arthritis Clinics
(medical scope interaction*)

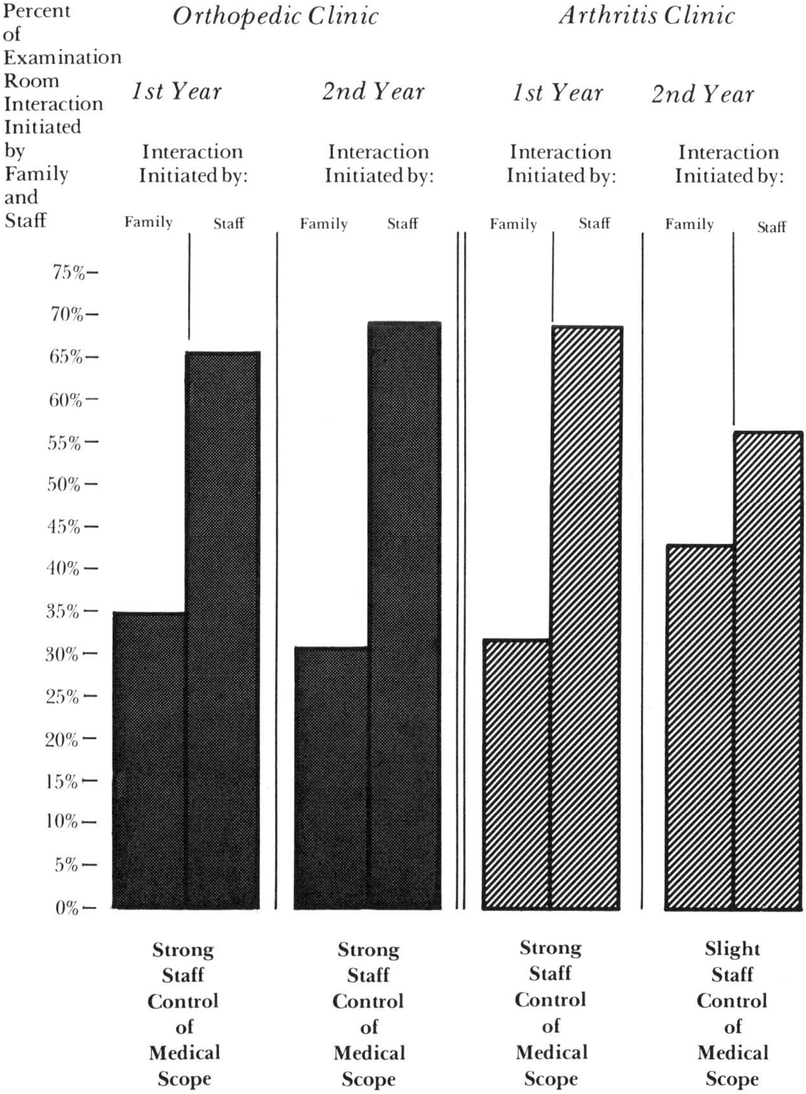

**Based on percentage data presented in Table II, Appendix B, pp. 202-3.*

GRAPH S-VII-9

Changes in Feedback Responsiveness* by Families and Staff in the Orthopedic and Arthritis Clinics

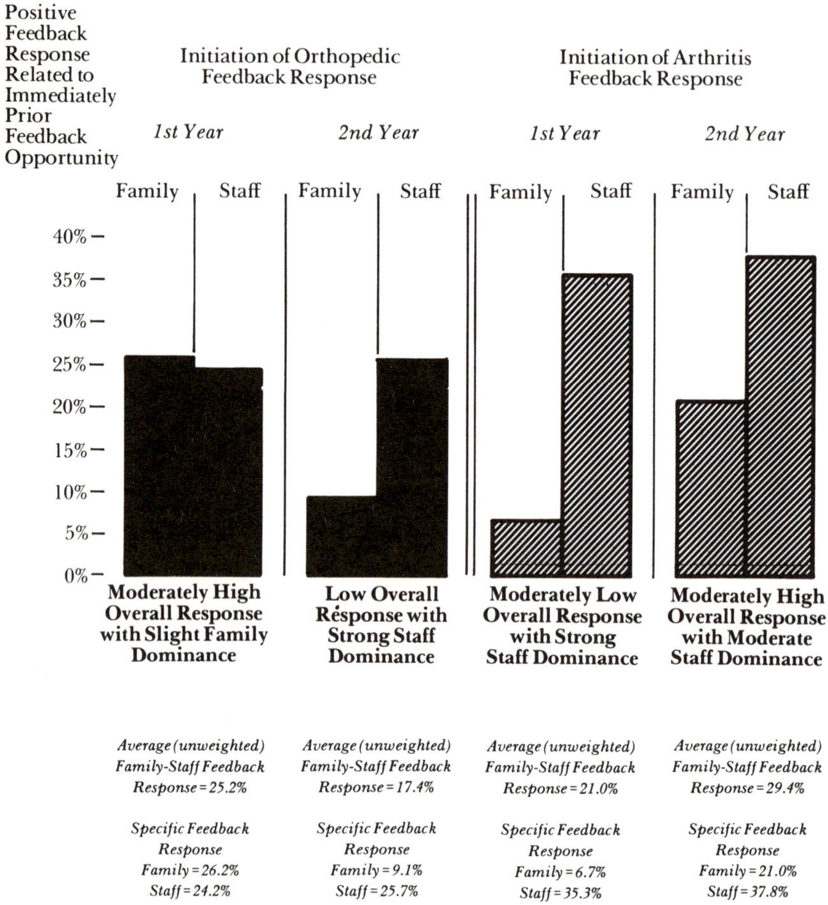

**Based on lagged regression analysis of data as presented in Table VI, Appendix B, p. 207.*

and decline of staff control of communication, trends which were opposite to those that took place in orthopedics.

A proximate factor in the sharp drop in orthopedic responsiveness was the increasingly rigid dominance of staff in medical scope in response to inquiries posed in home-related terms, by families. The failure of families to respond to inquiries in the new orthopedic clinic was traceable to the conflict between staff medical concerns and home-related interests of families.[25]

This discrepancy, though present in the first period of the research, was mitigated by a focused approach to family concerns through nursing mediation efforts. The administrative efforts of nursing to bend the hospital bureaucracy in the interests of families reduced the force of a medically dominated system. In the new building clerical personnel who took over from nursing the administrative operation of the clinic lacked the influence and experience to negotiate effectively for medical services to families who thus were left increasingly helpless in confronting the bureaucracy.[26]

VII-10. Declines in Flexible Coping Mechanisms and Support

During the prior year notable services were provided by the nursing staff in satisfying the needs of families, especially through its important administrative role of steering families through the bureaucratic maze of the outpatient department. Highly sensitive support was also provided to families with children suffering from scoleosis. The assurance and encouragement offered to these latter parents and children fulfilled an important need to trust the staff of the hospital, personified by the nurse, in facing the possible life-long problems of spinal correction. The relief shown by these parents and children was evidence of the important support contributed by the nurse.

In the new clinic administrative functions were delegated to clerical personnel, who were not able to fulfill the integrative leadership role of the nurse. The task of providing intimate support for families facing long-term scoleosis problems was organizationally separated from the orthopedic clinic. The loss of responsible, discretionary tasks in administration and primary health care signalled a rise in the non-mutuality of the cure orientation of a more impersonal professional approach to work.[27]

With the loss of non-routine functions, staff assumed a more "pro-

[25] For an example of this staff-family conflict over a medical versus home focus cf. above, a discussion of interaction in the arthritis clinic, II-8.

[26] This conclusion supports the finding of Terrien and Mills that the larger a service organization is the more time and money must be devoted to its administrative coordination. F. Terrien and D. Mills, "The Effect of Changing Size Upon the Internal Structure of Organizations," *American Sociological Review*, XX (February, 1955), pp. 11-13.

[27] The decline of mutuality in feedback patterns and staff rigidity in medical scope indicated a decline of persuasion and care functions as specified by Freidson. Increased non-mutuality signalled a rise in the cure orientation of esoteric professional work. Cf. Freidson, *Professional Dominance*, p. 120.

grammed" rather than "heuristic" approach to families.[28] Ritualized humorous forms of affect that had been important in releasing tension were replaced by routine forms of affective restraint. On the other hand, purely social contacts were fostered which had no evident connection with the continuing pressing demands of families for health services.

A key role in the integration of cure and care structures was withdrawn from the clinic by the nurse's withdrawal from administrative leadership. This disintegration of the clinic structure was signalled by the sharp decline of feedback responsiveness on the part of families. The decline of response by families during feedback communication indicated the disruption of the clinic as an adequately functioning setting for supportive activities.

With the withdrawal of nursing mediation in the interstitial areas, interactive rigidity increased and family responsiveness declined. A reasonably sensitive staff-based ritual coping institution became an increasingly defensive, structured and unresponsive health service.

[28] Ritual interaction, when used in primarily defensive ways as in the new orthopedic clinic approaches Thompson's "programmed-structure" rather than a "heuristic structure." Thus orthopedic staff response to family pleas was inhibited by a limited available repertoire of helpful interventions, while organizational pressures for many, rapid output transactions intensified "programmed" behavior. Cf. Thompson, "Organizations and Output Transactions," *American Journal of Sociology,* LXVIII (November, 1962), pp. 313-34. Cf. also Peter Blau, *The Dynamics of Bureaucracy,* Chicago: U. of Chicago Press, 1955, pp. 43 and 70.

CHAPTER VIII

THE CYSTIC FIBROSIS CLINIC: A FAMILY BASED RITUAL ORGANIZATION

As a coping support system, the cystic fibrosis clinic was in many ways an ideal type. More than any of the other clinics it was concerned with long range or life cycle issues. To a greater extent than in any of the other outpatient services a key role was played by health related community networks. Many families by virtue of their membership in local cystic fibrosis associations, showed a marked ability to cope with the problems of the illness and to deal with some of the impersonal procedures of the hospital. These families showed greater initiative in relating to the clinic staff, and hospital personnel displayed a more supportive attitude toward them.

VIII-1. Characteristics of the Clinic

The key role played by the cystic fibrosis association in encouraging family initiative and in gaining the attention of the staff was related to a number of special characteristics of the clinic. Of the illnesses treated in the four research clinics, cystic fibrosis was the most serious. Although the illness was frequently diagnosed early in childhood, there was no existing cure, the life expectancy being about twenty-one years. Moreover cystic fibrosis is hereditary in character. Among couples with family histories showing a proneness to the disease there is a high probability that their children will be afflicted by the condition. Thus, in the clinic, a feeling of guilt was evident in parental behavior toward the child. This was frequently expressed in the form of hostility directed toward the clinic staff, centering on deficiencies in hospital services. The behavior of clinic staff members also reflected depressed feelings stemming from the lack of medical control of the illness.

The approach of the clinic emphasized home management as long as the symptoms were not too grave. Periodic hospitalizations were required as flareups occurred, with hospital intervention increasing as the course of the illness progressed.

While diagnosis, examination and testing of children was controlled by physicians, most health teaching was carried out by the nursing staff. As in the diabetic clinic, the nursing staff used the waiting room for instruction in home treatment. Home care included rigorous control of diet, especially through low-fat cooking. Emphasis was also placed on medication, on respiratory exercises, and above all, on the use of the mist tent, to ease the child's breathing problems.

The behavior of the nursing staff during mist tent instruction was a remarkable feature in the cystic fibrosis clinic. The nurse explained the mist tent procedures in virtually the same words to each family that was contacted in the waiting room, even though these explanations were often of little use. In some cases, because of financial difficulty or poor family organization, there were no mist tents available. In other cases mist tent discussion did not fit family needs, as when mist tent cooling procedures were offered to families living where heat did not disturb the children's sleep. In other cases the failure of families to respond to the detailed explanations cast doubt on their ability to absorb and make use of these suggestions.

In interviews with the research staff, members of the nursing department explained that one of the difficulties confronted by the staff was the hostility of parents. The ritualized explanation of the mist tent seemed to be a way to deal with this hostility.

VIII-2. Role of the Cystic Fibrosis Association

Families that were active in the cystic fibrosis association were part of an on-going family community network[1] that fostered considerable self-help in dealing with the illness. They also benefitted from a base of emotional and technical support within the community in dealing with the hospital.

A definite pattern of behavior characterized these families' response to the ritual explanations of the clinic staff. They tended to redirect the rituals of the staff into channels consistent with their needs. Associa-

Cf. Elizabeth Bott, *Family and Social Networks.*

tion families often took over the interaction initiative from the staff and posed problems related to their own social situation. Staff members, though thrown off balance by this initiative, usually gave support to these home interests.

VIII-3. Care and Cure Centers in a Family Based Coping Organization

The cystic fibrosis clinic, as a family-based system, stressed home management of the illness. The use of the waiting room for health teaching, as in diabetes, reinforced this.

The head nurse enjoyed high prestige with physicians, as well as with other personnel in the outpatient department. She was well versed in the problems and dynamics of the illness and for several years had been in frequent contact with visiting families. The nurse confided to members of the research staff that as a matter of policy she tried to see every family in the waiting room for a few moments at the beginning of each clinic session. These brief contacts were used to assess new developments in the physical condition of the child and in emotional relationships within the family. These observations were used in conferences with physicians in the examination rooms before family interviews. They were also passed on to the social service department.

In contrast with the original practice in diabetes, physicians did not join the staff nurse in contacting families in the waiting room.[2] With no physicians present complaints could only be directed to the nurses. The absence of physicians also reduced the legitimacy of their activities there. The need for ritual explanations was intensified by this vulnerable position. Nurses tried to defend against this weakness by establishing contact with physicians in the examination rooms. The access of the head nurse to physicians, in the cure center of the clinic between family interviews, provided essential support for teaching activities in the waiting room. But the failure of physicians to enter the

[2] Rosengren and De Vault ("The Sociology of Time and Space in an Obstetrical Hospital, in Freidson, *The Hospital in Modern Society*, p. 271) point out the normative character of the segregation of activities in accordance with specific spatial arrangements. This normative element was supported by staff comments indicating the appropriateness of specific clinic areas for family contact. The avoidance of waiting room contact was justified in the surgical clinics by staff assertions of families' wishes to "have that door shut" in discussing their children's problems. In cystic fibrosis the nursing staff expressed the need to contact every family in the waiting room on their arrival in the clinic, for the purpose of noting family changes since the last clinic visit. Although the specific areas chosen varied from clinic to clinic, the normative preference of the staff regarding contacts with parents and children was quite definite in each outpatient service.

reception room constituted a failure to provide institutional recognition of the care center. The absence of this authoritative support intensified the mist tent ritual. (See Figure B-III-1, p. 34 above, for a general diagram of the clinic.)

VIII-4. Defensive Aspects of Mist Tent Rituals

The ritual explanations about management of the mist tent reflected the low technical control of the illness. The mist tent was not represented as a long range effective control of the condition of the child. Emphasis was placed on making the child more comfortable and better able to breathe and sleep, but no basic cure was offered. The emphasis on comfort suggested that the family should accept the inevitable course of the illness rather than expect a cure. The stress on home management and the slight attention given to treatment by drugs indicated the low reliance on medical technology by the staff.[3]

The repetitive, ritual behavior of the nursing staff underlined the non-specific character of their approach. Regardless of symptoms or needs families were uniformly exposed to the same patterned mist tent explanations. Families lacking active and effective social networks were completely passive during these ritualized presentations. Although in some cases they had adopted procedures suggested by the clinic staff, there was evidence that these suggestions were often ignored. The routine treatment prevented some families from raising issues that were bothering them and permitted the staff to avoid responding to complaints and anxieties that would otherwise have been raised.

VIII-5. Behavior of Association Families

This pattern of family passivity and staff defensiveness was absent when families were active in the cystic fibrosis association. The ability of these families to redirect clinic rituals was facilitated by several features of the clinic setting, among them the fairly small number of families at clinic sessions. Only about ten families attended each morning and afternoon of the week. Moreover, the chronicity and severity of the illness resulted in regular visits to the hospital. Over a period of time the families became familiar with the staff and their procedures. In particular, association families appeared to have developed counter-rituals in the form of specific activities in their local cystic fibrosis association. Reinforced by this social network these families were able to

[3] Evidence suggests that other medical systems tended to emphasize more intensive use of drugs and less reliance on mist tent care in dealing with the illness.

present individual problems that were bothering them and were able to alter the course of the institutionalized ritual patterns developed by the clinic staff.

VIII-6. An Example of Family Counter-Rituals

An example of the ability of association families to prevent clinic interaction from being dominated by staff ritual is presented by a family that was active in obtaining speakers for the local cystic fibrosis association. This family consisting of a father, mother, and a seven-year-old boy, was chatting with a nurse seated at a small table in the waiting room. Toward the end of the interaction the clinic nurse posed the following question to the mother:

Nurse to mother: Do you have any trouble with him . . . getting him too warm in his tent at night in the summer?

Mother to nurse: ummm . . . he doesn't complain, so we know about hanging some of those little ice things in the tent, but we thought if we once started it, he'd, you know, think it was something he had to have all the time and if he wasn't unhappy about the temperature of the tent—on a couple real bad nights, we have just left the tent up until the room has cooled off, and then we put it down.

Nurse to mother *(first words inaudible):* We live in the city area and it is going to be like this tonight when I go to bed too. It is going to be miserable. But some people, you know, if you live in a cooler area, it just doesn't bother the kids at all.

Mother to nurse: We put the fan on and pull the outside cool in and it almost always is, by the time we go to bed, cool enough, that, you know, we can have the mist tent down. I don't know there's any need to keep it cool, is there, unless he complains about it?

Nurse to mother: Just so he is comfortable.

Father to nurse: He doesn't have the sweating problem that some of the youngsters have, so this just doesn't seem to bother him much.

Nurse to parents: There is another thing too, that some parents won't put the child in the tent in the summer, because it is hot, so that is three months out of the year the child is not in a tent which isn't good for him. That is why I am trying to get everyone to know about this. They can put them in the tent no matter what. If you have any more questions about this, or if you think about anything or if I have anything to tell you, I'll . . . huh . . .

Mother to nurse: If you did the directions, I really would appreciate this, because we are going to have someone speak to our group who does work with machines (last words inaudible . . .), but you have some directions that he didn't have.

Nurse to parents: Okay.

Father to nurse: Thank you very much.

Nurse to parents: I'll show you what sort of directions I have, I've spilled coffee on them and every thing, but I'll—just as long as they . . . I get them back so I can type from them.

[Observer's comments: The nurse walks back up the corridor toward her desk area, looks through a folder, removes the typewritten form, returns back down the corridor . . . and she hands the form to the parents she had been talking with. As she turns to walk away, the nurse reminds the mother that this is the only typewritten sheet she has and asks her to return the form to her when they leave. The observer adds that this family belonged to "an organized regional group of parents of children with cystic fibrosis" and planned to use the information provided by the clinic nurse at a meeting at which a speaker would be discussing problems in handling the mist tent.]

This exchange illustrates this family's independence of some problems associated with the illness and its treatment. They succeeded in heading off the plan of the nurse to discuss cooling the mist tent. The family had adopted its own procedures, which were quite adequate and they needed no further explanations from the hospital. They did not want to become involved in a routine upon which the child might become dependent.

The family's involvement in organizational activities and dissemination of instructions to others in their community produced some insecurity in the nurse. She disclaimed ability to discuss the mechanics of mist tent operation and she referred them to the clinic technician. Her inability to represent herself as technically competent, and her referral of the matter to a non-medical technical expert, resulted in a decline in her authority with this family. This produced a change in the relationship between nurse and family, reflected in the character of the interaction at the end of the interview. Rather than have the nurse send the instructions on her own initiative to the family, the parents assumed the direction of matters by borrowing the clinic's material and making notes from them in preparation for the meeting which they were organizing.[4]

[4] The joint interaction of this father and mother suggests Bott's observation regarding the loose social networks of couples with joint conjugal roles. The reference to the association speaker who was unknown to the nurse indicated a

The change in relationship is symbolic of the coping behavior characteristic of association families. They came to the hospital with their own frame of reference and with a set of problems defined by a community network. Any initiative taken by the staff was responded to actively by these families in terms of their own socially shared experience. They did not passively react and accept the definition of the situation as provided by the clinic, but altered the content of communication to fit their own needs. They were able to reorient the ritual that the hospital had developed to deal with anticipated anxiety, guilt, and hostility. The association families were able to divert these ritualized patterns by developing counter-rituals of their own.[5] In this case the family was able to coopt the clinic nurse by using her as a resource for discussion at the local association meeting. The family also disrupted the image of the nurse as a technical expert and altered her impersonal offer of a mailed set of instructions.[6]

With the help of counter-rituals developed in their home community association families were not in need of the institutionalized coping devices constructed by the clinic.[7]

VIII-7. Authority Behavior and Ritual Patterns

Several features in this interaction reveal the role of ritual in the ac-

loose network approach in obtaining information from the hospital. Cf. Elizabeth Bott, *Family and Social Networks,* p. 59. The independence relative to the nurse also indicates Slater's concept of "role flexibility" wherein "everyone can play everyone else's role." Cf. Philip E. Slater, *Microcosm,* New York: John Wiley, 1966, esp. pp. 162 ff.

[5] These "counter-rituals" and family improvisation procedures appear to fall outside the classical Weberian bureaucratic model insofar as families cease to assume primarily passive roles in relation to staff. Cf. *From Max Weber: Essays in Sociology,* trans, ed. with intro. by H. H. Gerth and C. W. Mills, New York: Oxford Univ. Press, 1958.

[6] The behavior of this family in diverting the conversation toward getting help with their association activities suggests Scheff's analysis of the negotiating process between health personnel and patients. Cf. T. Scheff, "Negotiating Reality: Notes on Power in the Assessment of Responsibility," *Social Problems,* XVI (Summer, 1968), pp. 3-17.

[7] By pursuing their own objectives in a manner parallel to those of the nurse, this family was using the "conditionally cooperative strategy" pointed out by Solomon. Their independence in taking this approach was successful in altering the rather rigid pattern of the nurse to one of greater "cooperation". It appeared that this family was effectively coping with feelings of guilt and depression through this "conditionally cooperative strategy." Cf. L. Solomon, "Influence of Some Types of Power Relationships and Game Strategies upon the Development of Interpersonal Trust," *Journal of Abnormal and Social Psychology,* LXI (September, 1960), pp. 223-230.

tivities of the cystic fibrosis clinic. One aspect was the absence of reference, by either nurse or family, to staff physicians. Failure to mention physicians while they were absent from the interaction was a prominent characteristic of the clinic and was in sharp contrast to the behavior in the arthritis, diabetic, and orthopedic services. (This contrast with the other clinics is reflected by a quantitative analysis of the use of third person pronouns referring to physicians by mothers attending the clinic.[8])

The failure of families and staff to make reference to physicians in the cystic fibrosis clinic was most prominent during explanations of the handling of the mist tent, which were marked by no mention of doctors. Indeed during all passages of family interaction in which physicians were absent there were only ten references to them during the two weeks' activities of the clinic.[9]

The lack of reference to physicians by the nursing staff was related to the low level of medical control of cystic fibrosis. The mist tent explanations represented an effort to shift the responsibility for the care of the child to the family. The role played by the nurse in this effort was a key one. Their failure to refer to physicians was an effort to decrease reliance upon the medical staff and to increase family responsibility. This contrasted sharply with the arthritis clinic where, in spite of the uncertainties of the illness, emphasis was placed on dependency on physicians. The symptoms of arthritis could be ameliorated, if not eliminated; dependency on the arthritic medical staff was therefore encouraged.[10]

VII-8. Family Collective Expression

Family responsibility in the management of cystic fibrosis was displayed in the tendency to become collectively involved. This was reflected in the fact that fathers were more apt to attend clinic sessions and to participate in interaction than in any other outpatient service. Although he did not speak as frequently as the mother, the father's participation in the previous interview was crucial in controlling the flow of communication. The presence, and the verbal and non-verbal contributions of the father prevented the nurse from dominating the

[8] Cf. Appendix B, Table XIV.

[9] See frequencies and per line ratios for third person pronoun references to physicians while they were absent in the four clinics in Appendix B, Table XIV, Cols. 3 and 4. Thus in 2335 lines wherein the mist tent was not discussed there were 10 references to physicians, while no such references were made during 1497 lines of mist tent explanations.

[10] Cf. Appendix B, Table XVI, Col. 4, showing that physicians were referred to by third person pronouns once in every 18 lines in arthritis.

conversation and enabled the family to attain the goal they had set for themselves during the visit.

An empirical measure has been developed to explore the relative degree of collective expression on the part of families visiting the various outpatient clinics. If the four clinics are compared in terms of frequency of collective pronoun usage (as measured by first person plural pronouns used by mothers) the cystic fibrosis clinic had a much higher rate of frequency of collective expression than any other out-patient service.[11]

These collective forms of pronoun expression were most prominent in families that were active in the cystic fibrosis association. These families displayed a greater solidarity than those not active in the association.

VIII-9. Avoidance of the Child

A further feature stands out in the passages that have just been quoted. There was only one communication directed to the seven-year-old boy during the entire, rather lengthy interview.

The context of this avoidance of the child may be seen by comparing the cystic fibrosis clinic with the other outpatient services. Some of the clinics showed frequent communications with children attending the clinic. In the case of diabetes responsibility for care of the illness was placed very early in the hands of the child. This resulted in frequent communication, by both staff and parents, with children attending the clinic. To a lesser degree this was true in the orthopedic and the arthritis clinics, where children were required to assume a certain amount of responsibility for the management of their own condition. However, in cystic fibrosis, which is a degenerative and fatal disease, the child, particularly in his early years, was able to assume only minimal responsibility. Owing to the complexity of care it was the parents who assumed the bulk of responsibility. Thus fathers frequently undertook the construction of mist tent equipment.

VIII-10. Guilt and Avoidance Behavior

The failure of parents and staff members to interact with children especially during the mist tent explanations cannot be wholly explained on the grounds of technical responsibility. The pattern of interaction during these passages suggests that dynamic factors were at work. The child occupied the role of a tabooed person in the interac-

[11] Thus the line frequency average for each first person plural pronoun initiated by mothers was 30 in cystic fibrosis, 35 in scoleosis, 53 in arthritis, 74 in diabetes, and 118 in orthopedic. Cf. Appendix B, Table XV, Col. 6.

tion both to staff members and to parents. The fact that the mist tent made the child feel more comfortable and better able to sleep and did not cure or control the condition, was an underlying factor in the interaction.

The fact that the mist tent was attached to the bed of the child raised in various ways the issue of guilt. The fact that the child would have to continue to sleep in the tent for the rest of his life symbolized the fatal character of the illness. The mist tent symbolized the death bed of the child and raised the various culturally defined taboos associated with it. By avoiding the child, staff and families were able to deal with the mist tent as though it were not a tabooed object.

Unconsciously, the mist tent evoked the ambivalence of the parents toward the child as victim of the hereditary illness. By not referring to the child, and by treating him as a tabooed person, the guilt of the family was dealt with through avoidance.[12]

The failure to address children during the mist tent passages indicated the desire of the hospital to shift the burden of the child's care to the family. In that medical science had failed to develop an effective cure of the illness, the presence of the child in the interaction was a reminder to the staff of their medical failure. The tendency of the staff to address communication almost exclusively to parents was an attempt to avoid reference to that failure. The activities of this family in organizing regional meetings suggested that their mode of dealing with guilt was through denial. The avoidance pattern adopted by the nurse tended to reinforce this family method of dealing with guilt.[13]

VIII-11. Idealization and Association Families

While some association families dealt with guilt through denial, other families appear to have used idealization as a means of dealing with

[12] The treatment of the child through avoidance during the mist tent passages accords with Dumont and Foss's analysis of denial as basic to contemporary ways of dealing with death in America, especially with the death of children. Cf. R. G. Dumont and D. C. Foss, *The American View of Death,* Cambridge, Mass.: Schenkman Publishing Company, 1972.

[13] At the same time organizational activities whereby other parents were taught mist tent procedures, manifested conformity to the rules and commitment to the ideology of the cystic fibrosis association. This family by its conformity and commitment displayed the longitudinal and lateral biographical interests stipulated by Lefton and Rosengren for active client membership roles. In terms of these longitudinal and lateral interests these parents functioned as active clinic members in obtaining satisfaction of their needs from the staff. Cf. Lefton and Rosengren. "Organizations and Clients: Lateral and Longitudinal Dimensions," *American Sociological Review,* XXXI (December, 1966), p. 806.

this issue. This was the case with a family consisting of a father, a mother and a five-year-old girl. The observer commented that while the father was speaking with the nurse the child spontaneously threw her arms around him and said, "I like you." According to the observer the father smiled, as did the mother and nurse, at the child's show of affection. Following this exchange the interaction continued:

Nurse to mother: Does she have . . . mist in the tent?

Mother to Nurse: Yes.

Nurse to mother: How much fluid goes down in the bottle each night?

Mother to nurse: We use almost a whole bottle each night, except for maybe so much.

Father to daughter: Did you tell the lady you're the poster child?

Child to father: No.

Father to child: Why not?

Child to father: Cause, I don't know, I forgot.

Nurse to child: What did you forget?

Child to nurse *(haltingly):* I forgot I was, I forgot to tell the lady I was, um, that I was the poster girl.

Nurse to child: Are you the poster girl? Isn't that nice. You're a very, prettiest poster girls [sic] we've had, uh?

Child to nurse: Thank you.

Nurse to child: Oh you're welcome. [Father and mother laugh.]

Nurse to child: What are you doing this summer, are you having lots of fun?

Child to nurse: Yea.

Nurse to child: Do you go swimming?

Child to nurse: Yea.

Mother to child: Do you like to swim?

Child to mother: Yea.

Nurse to chitd: Where do you go swimming?

Child to nurse: It's a salt pond . . . . sometimes I don't even get, I don't even get a chance to get myself all wet.

Nurse to child: Really?

Child to nurse: Yea, I have to get my bucket and then . . . I have to get my bucket and get myself all wet with it.

Nurse to child: Well, at least you know, huh . . . How old are you now, Dorothy?

Child to nurse: I'm 5 and ¾.

Nurse to child: Are you going to go to school this year?

Child to nurse: My birthday is this summer . . . .

Nurse to child: You're going to be six, huh?

Mother to child: How old will you be?

Child to mother: I'll be six years old.

Nurse to child: You will be quite a big girl.

Child to nurse: I know.

Nurse to child: It's funny how you keep growing, isn't it?

Child to nurse: Yea.

Nurse to child: You're a bit of a riot sometimes, Dorothy.

Child to nurse: Yes.

Nurse to observer *(laughing):* Take that microphone away. Please don't stick the microphone in my mouth, I might bite down on it and get electrocuted.

Mother to child: You didn't tell her about the pool you've got or the name of your slide.

Child to mother: No, not yet.

Nurse to child: Well tell me about it, that sounds interesting.

Child to nurse: First, my mother and father couldn't . . . didn't know how to put it so we could slide in, when we put slide . . . when we put the slide on the pool.

Nurse to child: . . . then did you slide down the pool, slide . . . and land in the pool?

Child to nurse: Yea.

Nurse to child: That sounds like fun. That's lots of fun. It sounds like you're having a good summer.

Child to nurse: I know it.

Nurse to child: Good. See you later, Dorothy.

This interaction was very different from that with the previous association family. There was a greater desire on the part of the parents, particularly the father, to include the child in the conversation with the staff. Relationships were more tightly bound and openly expressed than in the previous case. This was reflected in the daughter's free expression of affection. Greater affective demonstration was shown when the father interrupted the conversation to invite the little girl to inform the nurse that she was poster girl for the cystic fibrosis association. The observer commented on the great charm of the little girl, who evidently had received considerable attention from her parents, particularly from the father. After this interjection about the child's role as poster girl, discussion of the mist tent, which had been initiated by the nurse, was completely replaced by attention given to the vacation activities of the child.[14]

This interaction involved basic social-psychological needs and mechanisms operative within the family structure. The attention given the child as poster girl and the unusual care devoted to her swimming activities suggested that the parents were attempting by focusing on the child's attractiveness to compensate for their problems.

As with the previous family the problem was how to deal with the guilt of the fatal and hereditary illness of the child. This family attempted to cope with the guilt by idealizing the child; this was accomplished by including her within the network of family activities and by making her the center of attention. Through this compensatory action the family diminished its guilt feelings, and the child, by playing the role of idealized person, contributed to this effort. The nurse, in giving her attention to the child during the clinic interview, reinforced this pattern of idealization and through it satisfied the need to assuage the guilt suffered by the family.

As with the earlier family the nurse's introduction of the mist tent discussion evoked the issue of guilt. Through their activities in the cystic fibrosis association this family brought its own approach to the problem of guilt. Through its participation with other association families idealization as a method for dealing with guilt was developed. When the nurse proposed the mist tent explanation the issue of guilt was raised, and the father enacted the family's mode of dealing with this issue.

In the cases cited, patterns of dealing with guilt were elaborated by the families themselves through the social network provided by their local health association. The hospital, by raising the issue of guilt in the context of the mist tent explanations, offered the opportunity for the family to reenact its own social-psychological life style in dealing

[14] The refocusing of conversation around home activities suggests Roth's observations on tuberculosis patients. Such persons are well informed clients who are apt to question and sometimes resist the actions and advice of staff. Cf. J. Roth, "The Treatment of Tuberculosis as a Bargaining Process," in A. Rose, *Human Behavior and Social Process*, Boston: Houghton, Mifflin, 1962, p. 577.

with the dynamics of the illness. The responses of the staff tended to reinforce the coping patterns that these families had developed.[15]

VIII-12. Role of the Waiting Room

Judged from the interaction in the outpatient department, membership in the cystic fibrosis association made families more active participants in a family-based coping system. With these families interaction with nursing personnel in the waiting room area was totally individualized. The use of the waiting room by the nursing staff created an appropriate setting for association families to present issues and understanding of problems that they had developed through contact with other families struggling with the disease. The opportunity to discuss these difficulties with the nurse in this family-based area put many families more at ease than in the examination room, where a restricted medical atmosphere prevailed. In this informal situation, with the less authoritative familiar personage of the nurse, parents were able to relax somewhat. In this more relaxed atmosphere they were able to claim some small success in combatting the illness.

VIII-13. Use of Examination Room for Acceptance of Illness

The clinic nurse enjoyed ready access to the examination rooms for contact with physicians concerning the progress of families. The opportunity to discuss families that had been interviewed in the waiting room served to reduce some of the strain on the nurse resulting from physicians' failure to leave the medical areas of the clinic.

Access to the examination rooms was also employed by the nurse for the purpose of confronting families more directly with the issue of acceptance of the illness. This practice was more prevalent with families that were not active in the cystic fibrosis association. These families frequently showed signs of disorganization and failure to perform the various tasks required in the treatment of the illness. With these families the nurse would present a more detailed analysis of the nature of the illness as a basis for achieving greater family responsibility. In the course of these discussions the issue of family acceptance of the

[15] The interaction with these families reflects aspects of the adaptive systems model proposed by Buckley. Thus a variety of responses was elicited in interaction by means of the mist tent explanations. Denial and idealization were verbally elicited as mechanisms by which families were coping with the illness. The staff tended to encourage active forms of these varied patterns and thus helped allay the guilt and ambivalence of parents. Passive and defensive forms of denial, involving neglect of the child, were confronted, however, during mist tent discussions in the examination room. Cf. Buckley, *Sociology and Modern Systems Theory,* p. 159.

illness sometimes arose. It appeared that the setting of the examination room was conducive to discussion of this delicate and distressing issue.

A typical case involving nursing interaction with families in the examination room is found in a passage involving a mother and seven-year-old boy. The father was not working, due to illness, while the child had to share a bedroom with the grandmother. The nurse initiated the interaction by inquiring about the family's use of the mist tent.

The sequence of interaction during this interview is very definite. The nurse first determined that the family was not using the mist tent. The mother gave as an excuse the crowded conditions in the home, and the illness and unemployment of her husband. The response of the nurse was to give a medical explanation of the value of the mist tent in clearing the lungs of the child. She explained further that ideally the child should spend all his time in a mist tent, but that this would be impractical:

Nurse to mother: Did I talk to you about mist tent care last time?

Mother to nurse: Yes you did.

Nurse to mother: How's that thing going?

Mother to nurse: Well, I haven't been using one of those tents.

Nurse to mother: That's right. When are you going to get him into a tent?

Mother to nurse: You see, I don't have the room right now. He really needs a room for himself.

Nurse to mother: Not really.

Mother to nurse: Well, his grandmother is quite old and that's noisy.

Nurse to mother: Do you have all the equipment?

Mother to nurse: I have the tank, is that what you call it?

Nurse to mother: The compressor.

Mother to nurse: Yes. And right now my husband has to go in the third of next month for a couple of operations and just as soon as that's all set, perhaps we can talk things over.

Nurse to mother *(understandingly):* Yes.

Mother to nurse: He's been out of work for a couple of months cause he doesn't feel well.

Nurse to mother: Well, it's pretty important that Thomas gets into one, you know. Do you know why we want him to get into one? Have we talked about that?

Mother to nurse: It helps more than the medication, right?

Nurse to mother: Well, it's this way, when you have cystic fibrosis—we all have mucus in our lungs.

Mother to nurse: Right.

Nurse to mother: I've got it, you've got it.

Mother to nurse: Right.

Nurse to mother: Right. The mucus in our lungs helps us clear out the dust, dirt, bacteria, and germs that we inhale all day long. Now, Thomas's is very thick and sticky—

Mother to nurse: Yes.

Nurse to mother *(continuing):* So it can't come out, it sort of sticks to the walls of the lungs and we can't get the dirt and the bacteria out. It blocks off things because it'll build up in that little tube, you know, and it'll stick to the walls again and again.

Mother to nurse: Yes, I think I've seen that displayed.

Nurse to mother: And the mist, you see what it does it liquifies it.

Mother to nurse: It loosens it up.

Nurse to mother: Yes. Now, if we could, we'd have all of our patients stay in the mist tent 24 hours a day. This way their lungs would work as normal as possible. Of course, this is impossible, we can't have some child walk around in a mist tent and try to go to school and everything. But when they're babies, we keep them in the mist tent longer.

Mother to nurse: Yes.

Nurse to mother: You can put them in the mist tent all day long because when they're up being fed and stuff. Of course, it's good.

Mother to nurse: Um.

Nurse to mother: That's as close to ideal as you can get. Of course, when the child is older, he has to be able to lead a life. You can't keep him in bed all day, that's for sure. He'll never get anything done, he'll never learn anything. But that's a—

Mother to nurse *(interrupting her):* It's just pitiful, that's all I think, really.

Nurse to mother: Well,—

Mother to nurse: Well, it's just unfortunate, really about these children.

Nurse to mother: Well, they lead normal lives though.

Mother to nurse: Sure.

Nurse to mother *(continuing):* I mean, uh, of course, they have to do a few extra things to lead a normal life.

Mother to nurse: That's it. Here they are on medication all the time.

Nurse to mother: There are a lot of kids on medication all day long, though, rheumatic, diabetic; all those things. [To child.] How are you doing?

Child to nurse: Lousy.

Nurse to child: You're doing lousy?

Child to nurse: Ah hah.

Nurse to child: Why?

Child to nurse: I don't know.

Mother to nurse: He's pulling your leg.

Nurse to mother: I know he is. [To child.] Yes, you're smart, huh? [Laughing.]

During this interview the mother interrupted the nurse to express her misery and sorrow at the plight of children suffering from the disease. The nurse replied by minimizing the condition with the assertion that with extra effort the child could have a reasonably comfortable life. The nurse also played down the severity of the illness by comparing it with rheumatism and diabetes. It is evident from these attempts to minimize the disease and from the bantering talk with the young boy, that the nurse judged that this family was not yet able to accept the gravity of the illness.

VIII-14. Examination Room and Acceptance of Mist Tent Use

It appears, however, that in some cases the examination room was effectively used in conveying to families the necessity of using the mist tent. Such was the case with adolescents who were more able to grasp the nature of the illness. The increased complexity of the disease along with social and emotional effects on the development of the child precipitated these discussions with families.

A conversation between the nurse and a family consisting of a mother and a young adolescent girl illustrates the successful use of the examination room for confronting the life-long need for the use of the mist tent. The nurse had previously explained to this family the mechanics of mist tent operation along with costs involved. This discussion had brought to light the social disruption to the child as a result of the installation of the mist tent in the bedroom. The observer commented that the young girl was noticeably upset by the damage to the bedroom furniture resulting from the spray produced by the mist tent. It is of interest that the family qualified under voluntary health insurance for a less expensive type of equipment. The more costly mist tent, which would not have been damaging to the child's bedroom, was not available under the insurance benefits.

In the following passage the observer introduced the remarks of the clinic nurse who explained why the hospital was providing a mist tent to the family:

[After a short time the nurse returned to the examination room and was followed by the mother and child who asked some further questions regarding the next appointment. At this point the nurse asked the mother and then the teenage child directly whether they had any other questions. The young girl appeared thoughtful for a moment and asked; "How long will I have to use this tent?" The nurse's answer was brief: "For the rest of your life," she said. The girl looked up at the ceiling and sighed but made no further verbal response. The nurse said that she knew it wasn't an easy adjustment and shared with the young teenager the feelings of another girl when she began using the tent after a number of years when (sic) she had not. The nurse continued as follows to the young girl:]

Nurse to teenage girl: . . . for the first time, and she noticed a big improvement. And now she wishes she had gone in it ten years ago when we told her to in the first place. Then she wouldn't do it. Or five years ago, or whenever we first tried to put her in a tent. It's just like anything else, when you . . . it's a prevention. It's just like when you were a baby, you had baby shots, so you wouldn't get diphtheria and you wouldn't get whooping cough and you wouldn't get things like this. You have your smallpox vaccination, and if you step on a rusty nail, you go get another tetanus shot. It's a prevention. If you think of it more like a prevention, it's not curing anything, because there's . . . you know . . . not curing anything because there's nothing . . . You feel fine, and there's nothing bothering you right now, as far as your lungs go. But it's prevention, to keep your lungs in the best possible shape you can. That's the reason we're giving it to you. Okay?

[Observer's comment: At this point the nurse smiled at the girl, who nodded quickly in response and the interview was concluded with the nurse and mother arranging the next clinic visit.]

The examination room was the location used by the nurse to urge the family to adopt the use of the mist tent. At no time during the operation of the cystic fibrosis clinic was this issue dealt with in the waiting room, even though the majority of interaction between nursing staff and families took place there. It is also of interest, as noted by the observer, that the nurse for the most part spoke directly to the mother. However, toward the end she did pay attention to the child and finally elicited from her a question which permitted discussion of the incurability of the disease.

The age of the girl was a factor that caused the nurse to seek an opportunity to discuss the gravity of the illness. The fact that she had entered adolescence meant that the illness inevitably would become more complex in its physical and emotional effects. At the same time the increased maturity of the child made it possible for the nurse to discuss the illness with mother and daughter, a circumstance which may not have been the case previously.

A number of social factors also magnified the problems. The first of these was the lack of involvement of the father. The weakness of the father's leadership in this family was reflected in his failure to assist in arranging for a mist tent and in the fact that the family was not active in the cystic fibrosis association. Membership in the association usually involved both husbands and wives, and it was typical for families that were active in the association to have both father and mother present during clinic visits.

The value of a network of families confronting similar problems is well illustrated by the issues that confronted this family. Among these problems were the economic questions involved in the obtaining of mist tent equipment. They could not afford the more expensive type of respiratory equipment described by the nurse. The more costly type of mist tent operated without damaging bedroom furniture. The prospect of this damage was especially disturbing to the adolescent girl.

Added to the economic problems of this family was the sheer complexity of the various steps required in managing the equipment and in providing treatment for the illness. Faced with this bewildering array of problems, many of which she could not grasp, the teenager was apprehensive and immobile through the greater part of the interview. The observer reported that the only time the child's expression changed was when the nurse was describing the tendency for the room and its contents to become sticky as a result of the mist tent spray. It may be inferred that the girl's loss of composure stemmed from her recognition that the mist tent would remove the image of a normal life that she had previously maintained to herself, her family and her friends. It was apparently anxiety about the disturbance of her life style that later led the child to inquire how long she would have to use the mist tent. Economic factors and limitations within the health system increased this family's stress and frustration and contributed to the disruption of their life pattern.[16]

VIII-15. Ritual and Acceptance of Death

In the case of families that did not become active in the association there was a lack of sufficient support structure within the home community for the parents to accept emotionally the inevitability of death. This failure of acceptance was demonstrated by the failure of non-association fathers to appear during clinic visits. Fathers who appeared in the clinic were also active in the association. When fathers of association families failed to attend, mothers and children were still very active in negotiating needs with the staff.

In those cases where the family lacked the community support structure to make possible the acceptance of the fatal illness of the child, it became necessary for the nurse as the most family-oriented person within the hospital to communicate to the child the need to accept his own death. The stress involved in attempting to communicate this directly rather than through the parents resulted in some of the extreme forms of ritual observed in the clinic.

It is thus possible to understand the use of ritual in the clinic through the pattern involving this family. In particular, the emphasis placed upon the mist tent comes into focus. During an earlier stage of the interaction the nurse inquired of the mother about the sleeping conditions of the family and learned that the child always slept under a blanket in the summer time since the nights were quite cool. Nevertheless, after a short digression, the nurse took up the procedure for cooling the mist tent through the use of frozen cans and a waste paper basket placed inside the tent. Although the nurse corrected herself later and recalled that the family had no need of these instructions, it seemed that she had a need to explain in full all of the procedures involving mist tent care. Although in this case, as with many other families, no discussion was included on diet or drug treatment, a complete coverage was offered regarding every aspect of mist tent main-

[16] It is of interest that, as the clinic nurse left the examination room with the mother and child preceding her, she turned to the observer and said that she was planning to leave the clinic. Her decision to leave the clinic was discussed openly with several other families in the context of friendly farewells exchanged with parents and children that the nurse had known for several years. It appears that the statement to the observer was, in part, a response to the stress that the nurse had been under during the course of this interview, a stress that stemmed from the need to confront this mother and daughter with the gravity of the child's illness.

tenance, the words following almost exactly the order in which they were presented to other families attending the clinic.[17]

This meticulous care in presenting every aspect of the handling of the mist tent was partly the result of the nurse's anxiety in preparing to confront this family with the incurable character of the illness of the child. In the case of families that were not active in the cystic fibrosis association the nurse faced the task of somehow convincing the child of the need to accept his own death. Thus the mist tent, as a symbol of the deathbed of the child, was to be used "for the rest of your life." The stress on mist tent care in all details was an effort to get the child himself to accept the inevitability of his own death from the disease.

The pressure involved in attempting to non-verbally communicate this acceptance was a great source of strain on the nurse.[18] With families lacking the support structure provided by the cystic fibrosis association this strain was increased by the fact that physicians spent most of their time with physical examinations and tests of the children and did not engage in much conversation with families. The burden of communicating acceptance of the disease to non-association families fell to the lot of the nurse.

By drawing this teenage child gradually into the discussion of the mist tent, the nurse was able to create an atmosphere for discussing the fact that the mist tent was "not curing anything." This remark was followed by the incomplete expression: "because there's nothing . . .", implying the incurable nature of the disease. To this suggestion some hope was added with a reference to the "prevention" the tent could afford.[19]

From the perspective of the analysis of ritual, the nurse assumed, for non-association families, the role of the absent father. (One might also add the role of the absent physician.) Through the explanations of the mist tent the nurse took on the guilt of the father and because of this guilt all emotional expression was repressed. The almost total absence

[17] A computer analysis is being done of these ritual patterns using a system of content analysis. The results of this study will be contained in a separate report.

[18] This pressure relates to the creation of "awareness contexts" as discussed by Glaser and Strauss. However, the role of ritual in these awareness contexts does not appear to be stressed in their analysis. B. Glaser and A. Strauss, *Awareness of Dying,* Chicago: Aldine Publishing Company, 1965.

[19] In terms of Wilkins' model of deviance, the mist tent ritual tended to amplify active forms of coping with the illness, while reducing passive, defensive procedures. The confrontation with this family in the examination room was aimed at reducing the passive avoidance of the fatal character of the disease. Cf. L. T. Wilkins, *Social Deviance,* Englewood Cliffs, N. J.: Prentice-Hall Inc., 1965.

of small talk and friendly efforts to involve the family and child in the discussion were typical of the mist tent passages. As a non-family member the nurse could not appropriately express the sorrow that grieved them at the future loss of their child. In addition there may have been repressed hostility against the parents for their failure to take responsibility in the care of the child. The ritualized explanations were aimed at inhibiting hostile feelings which the nurse felt for the parents' deficiency in assuming responsibility. The stress expressed in this family passage was also related to their inability to provide the best available mist tent equipment. Whereas in the orthopedic department of the hospital the finest technical resources were mobilized through the power of surgical medicine, the status of cystic fibrosis was less secure within the hospital structure and physicians were less able to implement the available medical technology. These institutional impediments combined with heavy stresses in confronting the guilt of families may have precipitated the nurse's decision to leave the clinic prior to the move to the new outpatient building.

VIII-16. Mist Tent Ritual and Support

In some ways the support afforded by the cystic fibrosis clinic is most evident with non-association families in which the issues posed by the fatal illness of the child were avoided. With a fatal, hereditary illness such as cystic fibrosis, the issue of acceptance of the death of the child was too crushing to be addressed directly. Acceptance of the illness and its fatal nature was indirectly approached by the adoption of mist tent care. The constant care by the family "for the rest of your life" gradually reduced the sense of guilt and induced a degree of acceptance of the fatal consequences of the disease.

In the case of cystic fibrosis association families the support structure of a community network assisted families in some degree in accepting the child's fatal condition. The support provided by the nurse was thus less demanding than with families lacking community network assistance.

Where families were isolated from community help, the support efforts of the nurse were most intense. As shown in the last passage the nurse almost directly stated that the mist tent was no cure for the condition of the child. By proposing the introduction of mist tent care, the nurse was putting forward the need for the family members to support each other in the acceptance of the child's death. The fact, however, that the treatment of this chronic illness is carried out primarily by the family itself made necessary a special kind of support by the clinic. By insisting on the family's obligation to take on the care of the mist tent the clinic, through the nurse, was offering firm encouragement for the parents and child to assist one another in accepting the fatal nature of the disease.

VIII-17. Location Use in the Cystic Fibrosis Clinic

The use of various ecological areas in the cystic fibrosis clinic paralleled, to a degree, that in the diabetes clinic. As in the latter clinic the nursing service functioned both in the waiting room and the examination rooms. In the case of cystic fibrosis more routine matters were handled in the waiting room. Here the nurse engaged in the structured presentation of mist tent procedures and in diet instructions. The nurse explained to the research staff that these measures were partly a defense against the hostility and frustration of families. In themselves, however, the mist tent instructions were also a method of diminishing the guilt of families by alleviating the condition of the children. By reducing guilt, indirect acceptance of the fatal illness was induced.

However, in more extreme cases with families that had not adopted mist tent procedures, or who were under severe stress because of the child's condition, the examination room became the scene of family interviews. There the nurse typically used the mist tent procedures as a means of opening up the issue of the gravity of the illness. As in arthritis the nurse used the medical atmosphere of the examination room to convey the serious, life-long character of the disease.

This need both for a routine setting and for a dramatized, authoritative location was reflected in the frequencies of area use in the clinic. Thus 87% of all family contact took place in the waiting room, while 8% occurred in the examination rooms. These figures reflected the incidence of relatively routine and more immediate, acute problems encountered during clinic sessions.[20]

VIII-18. Integration of Cure and Care Centers

As with the diabetic clinic, adequate delivery of nursing sevices to families required ready access both to the waiting room and the examination rooms. In cystic fibrosis, as in diabetes, the waiting room was the principal care center of the clinic. There the nurse conveyed to families an understanding of how they were expected to carry out their responsibilities in managing the day-to-day treatment.

However, since cystic fibrosis was an incurable illness, medical ineffectiveness, combined with the guilt of a hereditary disease, made contacts in the waiting room extremely stressful. In some cases when families displayed unusual hesitance in dealing with the illness, the

[20] The remaining 5% of family contacts occurred in the interstitial area of the administration desk. Cf. Appendix B, Ib. Such interviews with families tended to be brief, and were usually administratively oriented as in the orthopedic clinic. This percentage preponderance of the waiting room over the examination rooms as locus of family contact was greater than that recorded in any other clinic during both years' systematic observation periods. Cf. Appendix B, Table Ib.

nurse arranged to meet them in the examination room. Here she used the authority attached to the cure functions of medicine to impress on families the gravity and life-long nature of the disease. Without access to the cure center the nurse could not have performed the essential care function of conveying to families the need for acceptance of the child's long-term illness. The indirect approach to this issue by ritual in the care center, was reinforced by more direct treatment in the cure center.

VIII-19. Ritual Interaction and Affective Restraint

As seen from the interactions that have been discussed there existed a ritualized pattern associated with nursing repetition of mist tent explanations. Staff-family interaction took place in an emotional atmosphere of extreme restraint.[21] A distinctive feature of these interviews was the lack of fluctuation of feelings during the explanation of the various procedures. Relatively little variation in emotional expression occurred even during periods of more relaxed social contact. Nothing was observed similar to the frequent joking and small talk that occurred during periods of rest in the orthopedic clinic.

A computer analysis of affective behavior confirms the existence of this emotional restraint and invariance. A moderate level of feelings was evidenced during periods of low task activity, indicating a fairly positive amount of reserved affect.[22] During phases of more intense work activities feelings rose only slightly from this constant level.[23] Comparing the two modes of affective behavior, fluctuation in a measured tempo of feelings marked the pattern of interaction. This pattern suggested highly restrained interaction,[24] which differed radically from that observed in diabetes where wide positive predominance of expressed over reserved feelings took place. The pattern also varied sharply from that in orthopedic where reserved feelings were often dominant.

The contrast between cystic fibrosis and orthopedics as to affective patterning is shown in Graph T-VIII-19. Thus although overall levels of feelings were approximately equal in the two clinics marked differences in levels occurred in orthopedics, where feelings were used to relieve tension during non-work periods. In cystic fibrosis a steady

[21] Ritual processes as interactive patterns within coping systems are oriented to long range goals. This calls for a more restrained type of affect than is the case with rituals conducted in connection with short range crisis situations.

[22] (Shown by a reservoir ratio of 0.828). Cf. Appendix B, Table VII, Col. 3.

[23] Revealed by an expression ratio of 0.872. Cf. Appendix B, Table VII, Col. 4.

[24] Indicated by a slightly positive difference in affect ratio of +0.044. Cf. Appendix B, Table VII, Col. 5.

moderate "high" was maintained in both work and rest periods as a means of warding off the feelings of despair that pervaded the clinic.

The pattern of unwavering emotional restraint maintained through high and low work periods was appropriate to the ritualized interaction in the clinic. The fact that fairly intense feelings were sustained at

GRAPH T-VIII-19

Affective Behavior Patterns in the Cystic Fibrosis and Orthopedic Clinics during the First Year

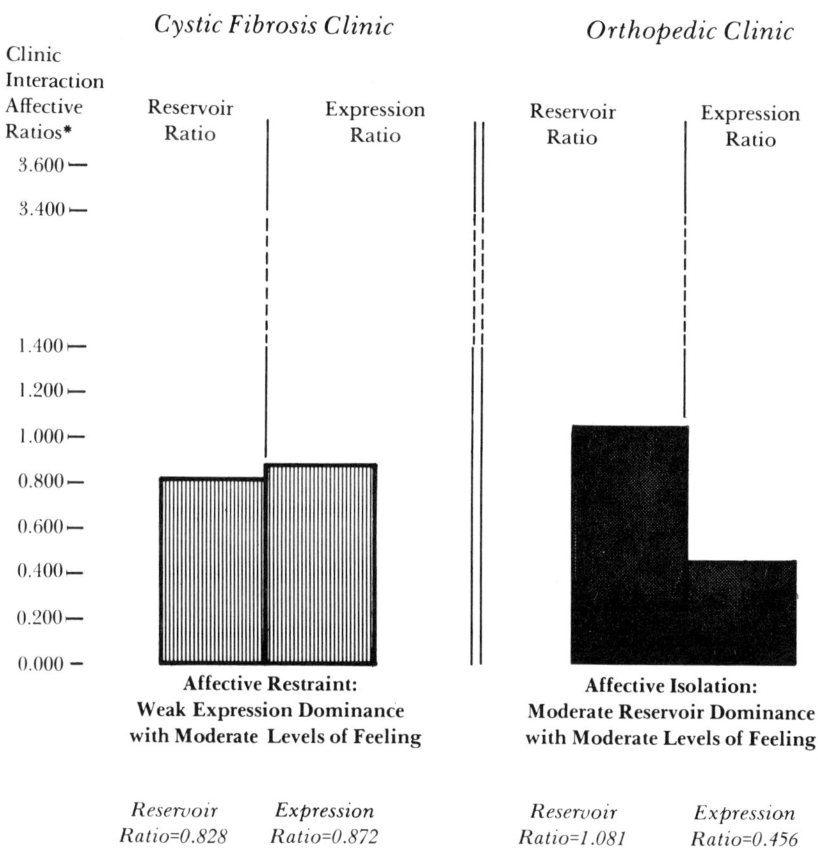

**Based on ratios presented in Table VII, Appendix B, p. 207.*

such a constant level throughout the interaction suggested the great affective investment of families and staff in the process.[25]

VIII-20. Ritual Interaction and Role Structuring

A correlation analysis of the four variables related to feedback process suggested a rather fixed structure of assigned roles in clinic interaction. With feedback and small talk assigned to family initiative, and feedback opportunity and courtship assigned to staff, sharp differences appeared in initiating patterns.[26] This difference was exceeded only once elsewhere in the course of the research (by the diabetic clinic during the first year).[27]

The sharp role structuring in cystic fibrosis contrasted with the reduced differentiation of interactive roles in the orthopedic clinic. This contrast is presented in Graph U-VIII-20, based on a correlation analysis of feedback related processes.

This rather precise structuring of family and staff interactive roles was consistent with the clinic as a ritualized network. Although association families tended to be involved in somewhat less rigid interactive roles, the depressed atmosphere tended to introduce rigidities in

[25] This observation would tend to support the view of Johnson and Martin on the dominance of expressive over instrumental components in the nursing role. However, the patterns of affect displayed in the various clinics suggest widely varying modalities of emotional feeling. Thuş in the first year of diabetes a "hard-sell" atmosphere of emotional diffusion prevailed with expressive highs during work periods accompanied by relative depletion of reserves. During the first year of orthopedics a climate of affective isolation prevailed accompanying a "soft-sell" approach. Here feelings were expressed outside of work-related passages as an expression of tension release (consistent with the task-group model—cf. T. Parsons and R. F. Bales, *Family, Socialization and Interaction Process,* New York: The Free Press of Glencoe, 1955). These affective patterns are within the culturally prescribed norms of western industrialism. The pattern of constant fairly intense emotional expression (described as "restrained") during both work and non-work situations is beyond existing cultural norms. It is associated with the attempt of nurse and families to overcome depression due to guilt and ambivalence. It may be regarded as a hyper-normal "high", and as such is an affective coping mechanism for dealing with the problems faced by cystic fibrosis families. Cf. M. M. Johnson and H. W. Martin, "A Sociological Analysis of the Nursing Role," in H. M. Vollmer and Donald L. Mills, eds., *In Professionalization,* Englewood Cliffs, N. J.: Prentice-Hall, 1966.

[26] As shown by an overall correlation difference of +1.541. Cf. Appendix B, Table IV.

[27] Cf. Appendix B, Tables IV and V.

GRAPH U-VIII-20

Role Structuring in the Cystic Fibrosis and Orthopedic Clinics during the First Year

(medical scope interaction*)

Cystic Fibrosis Clinic *Orthopedic Clinic*

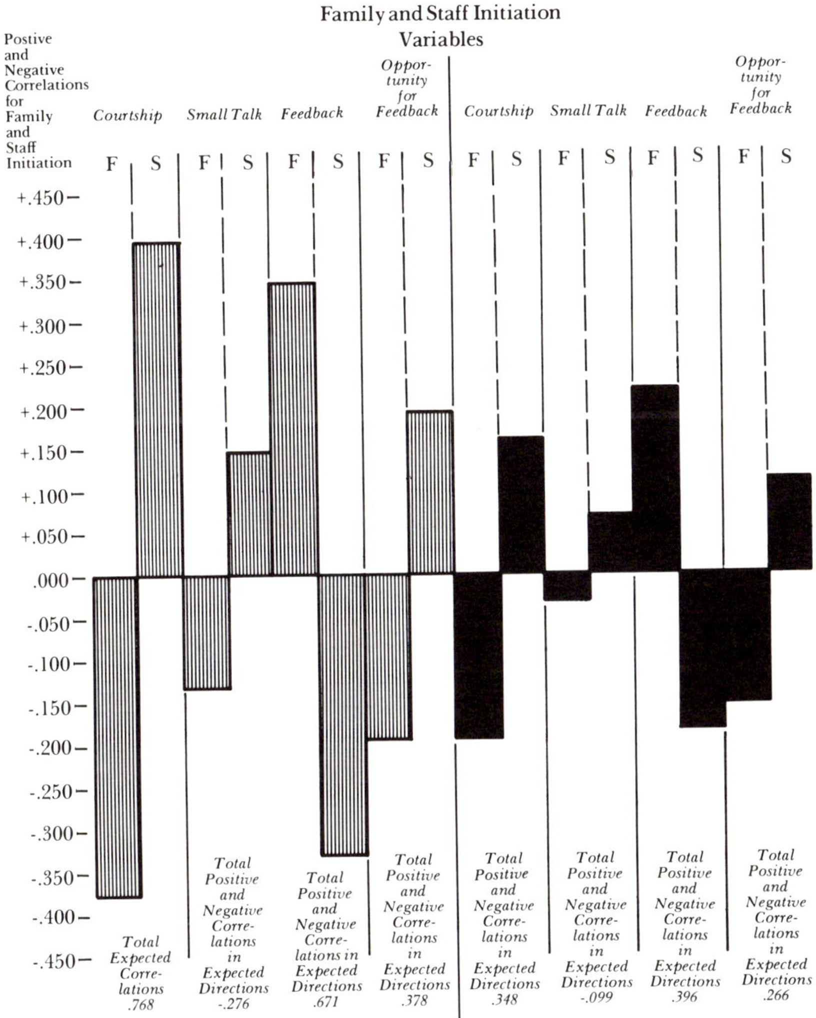

Moderately High Structuring: Overall Total of Expected Positive and Negative Correlations=1.541

Low Structuring: Overall Total of Expected Positive and Negative Correlations=0.911

Based on lagged correlations as presented in Table IV, Appendix B, p. 205.

role assignment. The contrast here was greatest with arthritis where flexibility of interactive structure was the rule.[28]

VIII-21. Ritual, Medical Scope and Staff Initiative

Consistent with a conceptual pattern of ritual interaction, activities between staff and families were concentrated at medical scope and tended to be staff dominated. Thus 63.6% of all interaction was initiated by staff members, while 89% of the content of the activities was medical or technical in nature.

When staff-family initiation is compared by scope and location, families were considerably more active in waiting room than in examination room sequences. This difference accorded with the use of the waiting room for more routine matters (suggested by a 34.4% family medical scope initiation), while more grave concerns relating to acceptance of the illness were discussed in the examination rooms (indicated by a 22.9% family medical scope initiating rate[29]).

This pattern was not consistent with examination room activities in the diabetic clinic and in arthritis[30] where families were often noticeably more active in the examination rooms than in other locations. The issues of acceptance of the illness and death of the child were associated with the depressed rate of family initiative in the cystic fibrosis examination rooms.

VIII-22. Intense Feedback Responsiveness

This configuration of affective restraint, fixed interactive structure, low family initiative, and medical emphasis produced a ritual pattern generated by the dynamics of family guilt, depression and ambivalence. Along with this well defined structure the cystic fibrosis clinic attained the highest combined feedback responsiveness recorded in the course of this research. A high staff feedback response of 34.0% and a comparably intense family response to feedback opportunity of 25.7% produced an average rate of 29.9%. This combined percentage even exceeded that achieved by the sensitive feedback interaction developed in the arthritis clinic during the second research period.[31]

This high level of sensitivity and willingness to reply to inquiries is surprising given the structured and ritualized patterns in the clinic. It appears that the intensity of replies to requests for feedback was due to

[28] Cf. Appendix B, Table IV, indicating that the arthritis clinic in the second year showed a difference in role structuring of 0.782.

[29] Cf. Appendix B, Table II.

[30] Cf. Appendix B, Table II.

[31] Cf. Appendix B, Table VI, showing an average rate of feedback response in arthritis of 29.4% (based on an unweighted average percent).

the focused approach adopted by the clinic nurse to the problems of family grief and guilt.[32]

Graph V-VIII-22 indicates a higher overall feedback response level in cystic fibrosis than in the orthopedic clinic. Thus the ritualized structuring of roles and steady "high" intensity of feelings produced a highly responsive feedback process. On the other hand, despite less structured interaction and a freer mode of overt feelings, a lower feedback response was achieved in the orthopedic clinic.

The mist tent passages addressed the underlying ambivalence and grief of the parents. By adopting the mist tent care of the child, the parents could do whatever was possible to make the condition more tolerable. In so doing they could reduce their own guilt and gradually induce acceptance of the fatal character of the illness.[33]

With families who were members of the cystic fibrosis association, the mist tent expositions raised the issues of ambivalence and acceptance and provided opportunities for the initiation of counter-rituals. Mist tent passages evoked exchanges about the families' community coping methods. While this redirection of discussion sometimes unbalanced the nurse, the invariable result was a sensitive feedback exchange.

With non-association families, the mist tent passages often raised the question of acceptance of the illness. In this way mist tent discussion was used by the staff to sensitize families that attempted to avoid the issues of cystic fibrosis. The focused use of this ritual evoked intense and tragic feelings, but in a significant number of cases resulted in a meaningful feedback exchange on basic issues.

VIII-23. Ritual and a Longitudinal Family Based Supportive Organization

Systems may be distinguished by their tendency to deal or not to deal

[32] The presence of high level of feedback sensitivity in a structured, ritualized interactive network seems consistent with Hall and Fagan's analysis of static and dynamic systems. In cystic fibrosis a static focus was assumed on the issues of guilt and ambivalence of parents. Ritual treatment of these issues evoked feedback from parents in their efforts to cope with the children's illness. These efforts by the parents to cope with the children's illness received feedback support from the nurse. Cf. A. D. Hall and R. E. Fagan, *Definition of System,* New York: Bell Telephone Laboratories, 1956.

[33] Roth maintains that in the case of contagious illnesses ritualized procedures are for the convenience of administration. In the case of hereditary, fatal children's illnesses focused ritual may have a function in overcoming fear, grief and ambivalence. Cf. J. Roth, "Ritual and Magic in the Control of Contagion," *American Sociological Review,* XXII (June, 1956), pp. 310-314.

GRAPH V-VIII-22

Feedback Responsiveness*
by Families and Staff in the
Cystic Fibrosis and Orthopedic Clinics
during the First Year

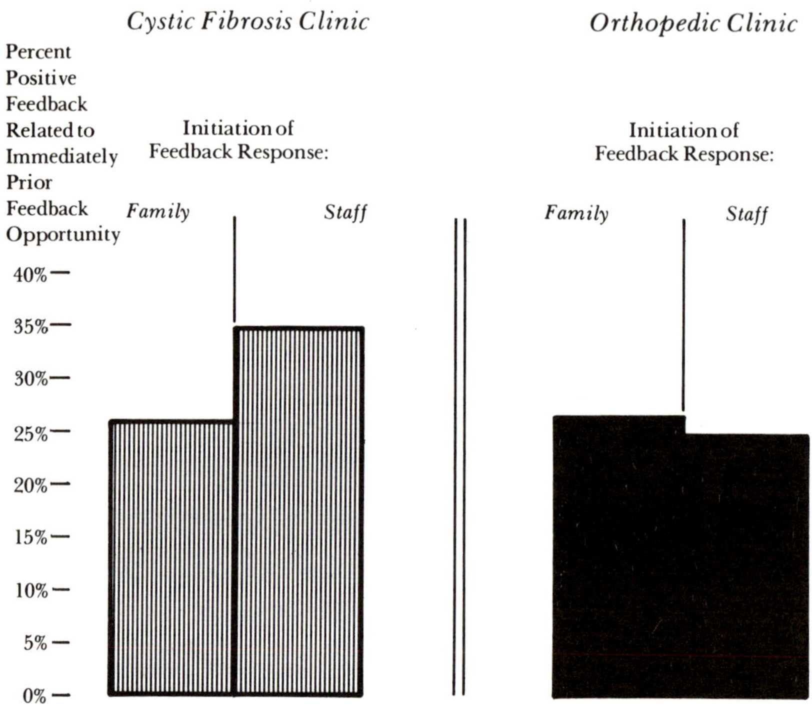

Cystic Fibrosis Clinic	Orthopedic Clinic
Moderately High Overall Response with Moderate Staff Dominance	**Moderate Overall Response with Slight Family Dominance**
Average (unweighted) Family-Staff Feedback Response=29.9%	*Average (unweighted) Family-Staff Feedback Response=25.2%*
Specific Feedback Response Family=25.7% Staff=34.0%	*Specific Feedback Response Family=26.2% Staff=24.2%*

**Based on lagged regression analysis of data as presented in Table VI, Appendix B, p. 207.*

with longitudinal dimensions of the life-space of their clients.[34] The appearance of ritual in the context of integrated use of the care and cure centers established the cystic fibrosis clinic as a longitudinal system. By ritual use of the mist tent, guilt of parents was reduced and acceptance of death was fostered. The ritual pointed to the need to maintain this focus longitudinally for the life-time of the child.

The symbolism of the bed and the mist tent around it expressed both the death bed of the child and the marital bed of the parents. This symbolism both expressed the ambivalence of the parents toward the child and offered a practical means of reducing these ambivalent feelings.[35]

The integration of the cure and care centers of the clinic, therefore, was achieved by ritual as a central institutional mechanism in a family-based coping system dealing with guilt and the acceptance of the premature death of children.

[34] M. Lefton and W. R. Rosengren, "Organizations and Clients: Lateral and Longitudinal Dimensions," *American Sociological Review*, XXXI (December, 1966).

[35] Cf. J. Rheingold, *The Mother, Anxiety and Death:* the catastrophic death complex. Boston: Little, Brown, 1967.

CHAPTER IX

THE CYSTIC FIBROSIS CLINIC: CHANGE IN A FAMILY BASED RITUAL ORGANIZATION

The changes that occurred in the cystic fibrosis clinic were of a different quality than those in any of the other clinics. The large brightly colored new waiting room, wide corridors and tastefully furnished examination rooms all had a cheering effect on families attending the clinic. There was an effort on the part of the nursing staff, physicians and auxiliary personnel to hearten families and especially children during clinic visits. The waiting room area was equipped with blackboards and colored chalk, with low tables and children's chairs, used by nurses and auxiliary staff to engage the children in play while waiting for clinic services. Physicians were also more relaxed in the new examination rooms and spent time in socializing and in attempting to get children to feel more at home. The staff was quite happy with the new quarters and wished to make as good use of them as possible in the service of families. The expansion of the medical areas enabled physicians to spend more time individually with families, and the increase in laboratory facilities and private physicians' offices had a positive effect on the morale of the medical staff. In addition, a large nursing station was provided for the head nurse and her assistant; the area was used as a place of retreat by the nurse when the stress of clinic activities became too great. (See Figure C-III-1, p. 34 above.)

In addition to the greater comfort, improved decor and generous size of the clinic, the staff also was increased. Another full-time resident was added, so that in addition to the chief, who remained in charge of operations, there were usually four physicians on hand to attend an average of 25 families during the daily sessions of the clinic.

A social worker was in regular attendance during clinic sessions and was active in contacting adolescent patients whose adjustments to the complexities of the illness were very stressful. A physical therapist was added to the staff to assist with special problems when they arose.

The nursing staff also underwent significant changes. Prior to the move the head nurse who had been serving in the cystic fibrosis clinic discontinued her connections with the hospital. Her place was taken by a younger colleague whose task it was to assume the burdensome duties of assisting families and maintaining contact with physicians and other personnel.

The new head nurse was less experienced in the problems of cystic fibrosis and particularly in the dynamics of the illness as it affected family relationships and behavior. She was handicapped by personal unfamiliarity with client families and their individual physical, psychological and social difficulties. She lacked the close staff rapport, especially with the chief, that the previous nurse had developed. Although the previous nurse had borne great stress in dealing with emotional problems of families and technical difficulties of the clinic, she had enjoyed the respect of the chief and other members of the staff, which had made these strains more tolerable. While she had frequently shown extreme anxiety and isolation in attempting to cope with the guilt and ambivalence of families, she had received personal encouragement from physicians on the staff. This support was lacking in the form of public legitimizing of her efforts through failure of physicians to appear during teaching sessions in the waiting room, but she had enjoyed free access to clinic examination rooms. There she had reviewed with physicians the health and behavior of children and parents which she had observed during waiting room conferences. She had had access to examination rooms for individual contact with families, and had made use of these contacts to assist them in confronting the acceptance issue. The mist tent ritual had facilitated the emergence of this issue during these contacts.

IX-1. Discontinuance of Mist Tent Rituals

During the second year, the new head nurse discontinued this focused, ritualized approach to mist tent exposition in family interviews. She concentrated on making children feel more at home in the clinic setting. Considerable time was spent playing with children and attempting to get them to smile and engage in playful conversation both with physicians and with other members of the clinic staff. In some cases she was successful in getting the child to relax and accept the unfamiliar environment of the new outpatient building. It was difficult to assess the long term value of this effort, but it may be surmised that some success was achieved in reducing children's anxiety in relation to the unfamiliar, threatening hospital situation.

The approach to parents attending the clinic sharply contrasted with that of the previous nurse. The emphasis in contacts with families, which often took place in the waiting room, was either on the social aspects of the home situation of the family, or on efforts to cheer up the parents. The efforts of the nurse to discuss non-health related issues met with chilly or hostile response. Families appeared to be under great stress and were not inclined to discuss problems that were not related to the condition of the child.

Efforts of the nurse to encourage parents about the physical condition of their children appeared to lack an adequate reality basis. The encouragement offered arose more from the anxieties of the nurse attempting to deal with the stressful situation than from any focused and organized effort to calm family fears. These difficulties were compounded by the fact that she was relatively unfamiliar with some medical aspects of the illness. The tendency to bring up the use of drugs contrasted with the practice of the previous nurse who avoided areas of strictly physician concern.

This change in personnel and consequent redirection of emphasis is a rather cogent commentary on nursing training. The new nurse exhibited normal human instincts in refocusing her efforts and abandoning the mist-tent ritual. Her activities were directed more toward the anxiety of the child and toward making the clinic visits "pleasant" for the family. These immediate goals took precedence over the long range supportive goals of her predecessor. If the effectiveness of the ritual had been recognized as the strength of the support function it most certainly would have been continued. This could have been accomplished, however, only through a program of ongoing retraining in the nursing profession.

IX-2. Removal of Ritual as Coping Mechanism

The abandonment of the ritual presentations of mist tent care as a means of dealing with the acceptance issue deprived the nurse of an important authority function as mediator of stress and alleviator of family guilt and depression. The ritual explanations had offered means by which parents could assume responsibility for their children and so diminish guilt and increase acceptance.

Insofar as the first nurse had assumed the guilt of parents' inability to provide adequate care for their children, she had assumed a part of the authority of the parents. To the extent to which she had replaced the physicians during the ritualized explanations of the mist tent, she also had taken on her shoulders the failure of medicine in not achieving an effective cure. The first cystic fibrosis nurse had therefore been in a position of high symbolic authority. This dual assumption of parental and medical authority had given her considerable informal leadership both with families and with members of the staff. A number of families expressed their strong feelings of disappointment to the nurse when she told them of her plans to leave the hospital. The integrative role of the nurse as alleviator of family and staff feelings of inadequacy was lost to the clinic through her departure.

IX-3. New Nursing Approach to Family Problems

The effects of this loss to the integrity of the clinic as a supportive coping institution are evident from an interaction with the mother of an older adolescent child who was anxious about the increased physical and emotional problems of her daughter. She expressed her fears about the child's weight loss, nausea and fever. The daughter was nervous and irritable, and the mother expressed some guilt that the child had not been taking all her medicines. More recently the daughter had been following all the medical directives by sleeping in the mist tent, doing physio-therapy and faithfully taking the drugs prescribed by the physician. The mother expressed concern that the child was not doing well despite her observance of the medical regimen.

The mother then took up the difficulties her daughter had been having in contacting clinic doctors.

Mother to nurse: . . . and, of course, she got disturbed because Dr. Evans told her the last time she was here, that if she didn't feel well to give a call, and he would talk to her. She tried three times and couldn't get Dr. Evans.

Nurse to mother: I know.

Mother to nurse: Last time she called she got Dr. Quinn and he wasn't ready to listen to her. He just asked for her phone number and said that he would have Dr. Evans call and he had never called. So if he left a message at home I don't know but this really bothered her.

Nurse to mother: You know in a situation like that I wish that I had known about that. Because I would have been able to get through to somebody.

Mother to nurse: Um . . . Well this morning . . . told her. . . .

Nurse to mother *(interrupting):* Because Dr. Quinn is supposed to be there and he. . . .

Mother to nurse *(interrupting):* In fact she even asked if I called him. Well, I certainly will, well I'll get someone, I don't care who calls you up. Otherwise when we called up we talked to Dr. Royce and Dr. Carlton. So that we can get Dr. Carlton . . . but, uh, as I say, I was determined to get somebody! But apparently she didn't . . . or say enough about herself, you know, for what I don't know . . . . because she did not get a hold of Dr. Evans.

Nurse to mother: You see the doctors, for example, are sometimes on call on the wards or sometimes making rounds . . . and, uh, if we leave a message with the secretary the same thing is going to be bound . . . even if I gave you for example, a phone number. But, I am here . . . pretty much most of the time during the day. So if it were difficult to find a doctor, you know, you could try me. And though it were difficult and though I couldn't do anything, I would know where to go.

Mother to nurse: . . . But you know, she feels nervous about letting them know . . . so that in her mind when she called she wanted to talk to Dr. Evans. . . .

Nurse to mother: She gave up.

Mother to nurse: That's why, as I say, I called the department and I didn't care who I talked with. If I have to talk to Dr. Carlton I'll talk to him. To begin with . . . as it turned out Dr. Evans . . . . [mother laughs]

Nurse to mother: Well how many . . . good. Do you think it would be good, to have . . . . [my] number, would that help? Do you feel . . . .

Mother to nurse: *(interrupting):* . . . who knows what might happen . . . .

Nurse to mother: *(interrupting):* . . . do you think that would be just . . . order. . . . value . . . .

Mother to nurse: If I can get someone. . . .

Nurse to mother: Let me give you my number.

Mother to nurse: Sure.

Nurse to mother: Okay . . . my number . . . and if you can't reach Dr. Evans . . . .

Mother to nurse: I haven't got your name . . . . I never can remember your name.

Nurse to mother: I know it. Nobody can . . . and I don't remind them sometimes. So that . . . that doesn't help people but let me get a piece of paper. [Nurse leaves and returns in a short time with paper and pencil.]

The problems of this family presented special difficulties to the staff. The anger and frustration of this mother had a basis in the worsening physical and emotional condition of her 18-year-old daughter. The serious condition of this girl, as indicated by her symptoms was a cause for constant worry. Moreover there was no one else in the home to supply support to the mother in these trying circumstances. The family situation was complicated by financial problems; the daughter was no longer working and was drawing unemployment compensation. There was also evidence of extreme psychological stress reflected in great tension between mother and daughter and by the daughter's unwillingness to discuss her condition with anyone except her own physician. The strain on the mother was evident in her repeated interruptions of the efforts of the nurse to offer help.

Problems of this kind were not absent from family interviews during the first year in the cystic fibrosis clinic. It had not been uncommon for families to complain about their failure to contact a physician by phone. As in the present instance the nurse would offer to provide a phone contact for the family to place them in touch with the physician in charge of their case.

Despite the serious problems of this family, the behavior of the staff suggested a serious defect in the operation of the clinic. Following the physician's instructions that she call if she felt ill, the daughter tried three times unsuccessfully to reach her physician at the hospital.[1] The mother's intervention apparently further increased the tension of the daughter, which was evident in the moody manner she displayed during the visit.[2]

[1] Despite the ambivalence evidenced by this mother toward her daughter's emotional behavior, there was resentment expressed toward the physicians for their failure to respond to the family's requests for help. This resentment, which was shared by the daughter, is related to Haug and Sussman's analysis of the revolt of the client against professional and organizational autonomy. Cf. M. R. Haug and M. B. Sussman, "Professional Autonomy and Revolt of the Client," *Social Problems,* XVII (Fall, 1969), pp. 153-161.

[2] The rise in tension and in family hostility toward the hospital may be related to Leavitt and Mueller's observations concerning effects of "zero feedback". Under experimental conditions zero feedback engenders hostility, which is perceptible when conditions of free feedback are instituted. Existing tensions within this family were intensified by the failure of the hospital to respond to calls. These tensions were expressed as hostility, partly toward physicians during free feedback with the nurse. Cf. H. Leavitt and R. Mueller, "Some Effects of Feedback on Communication," in Hare, Borgatta and Bales, eds., *Small Groups: Studies in Social Interaction,* pp. 414-423.

IX-4. Causes of Clinic Communication Problems

The difficulties experienced by the clinic in responding to the problems posed by this family point to structural difficulties that emerged with the move to the new building.[3] In the old clinic, although the nurse was primarily concerned with instruction relating to respiratory and diet problems, a close working relationship was also maintained with the clerical staff at the administration desk. It was the practice of the nurse in the old clinic to distribute cards to families dealing with various tasks required during clinic visits. This procedure was used as a means of checking on recent developments within the family. This administrative work also kept the nurse in touch with the clerical staff with whom she would often arrange new appointments for families. Due to the close cooperation between the clinic clerk and the head nurse, in unusual cases such as that of this family, contact between the patient and the child's physician was usually maintained. The failure to respond to acute family need that occured in the new cystic fibrosis clinic was unparalleled in the other outpatient services during the course of the research.[4]

The failure of communication, which was not a unique occurrence in this clinic during the second year, resulted from the disappearance of an integrative nursing function within the clinic structure. The immediate cause of this failure was the inexperience of the nurse with the illness and her unfamiliarity with parents and children.[5]

IX-5. Loss of Nursing Integrative Role

The new nurse was not in the position to offer the kind of dominant leadership that was apparent in the first year of the research. Authori-

[3] This was somewhat reminiscent of the problems that arose in the course of the move of the orthopedic clinic, a difficulty traced to new administrative arrangements.

[4] The ineffectiveness of the clinic in responding to the acute problems of this family suggests the dangers of specialization and fragmentation of ambulatory outpatient care in which, according to Freidson, the patient feels little continuity of attention. Cf. E. Freidson, "Organizing Ambulatory Medical Care," in *Professional Dominance,* p. 197.

[5] The nurse attempted to relieve the mother's guilt by saying "You have done all you can." This remark evoked the dispairing response that she had done all she could and still the child was not improving. This feeling needed to be expressed, but the mother was also in need of assurance that if she called the nurse assistance from the medical staff would somehow be arranged. An essential nursing role as intermediary in interpreting the crisis needs of families to physicians was brought out through the difficulties faced by this mother and daughter.

tative leadership could only be achieved in this clinic by dealing with the feelings of guilt and depression underlying the behavior of staff and families. These issues were handled in the first year by the head nurse through the ritualized mist tent explanation. Through this mechanism she conveyed to families, especially parents, the basic incurability of the condition. By dealing with the issues that were central to both families and staff, the nurse had become the appropriate integrator of the clinic as a coping system.

IX-6. A Family Based Coping Institution[6]

The clinic, as a supportive institution, was family-based. The use of the waiting room and adjacent interstitial areas for contact with families continued at a somewhat diminished rate. During the first year such public areas absorbed 92% of family contact[7] and during the second year family contact there declined to 65%. The clinic still far exceeded the staff-based surgical clinic, in the use of public areas for family contact and was almost on a par with diabetes (with 76%).[8]

This emphasis on public area use was associated with continued efforts to underline family responsibility for the management of the illness. In the new location stress was placed on nursing instruction on diet and medical treatment. The abandonment of the mist tent ritual and the consequent disruption of symbolic coping processes brought about a decline in various quantitative and qualitative indices of health service delivery.

IX-7. Administration and Negative Trends in Family Service

The qualitative analysis pointing to a decline of the ability of the clinic to cope with the family anxiety is supported by quantitative indices from the data. A comparison of all the interaction for two years shows that nursing interaction with families decreased from 62.0% to 45.3%. This decline of 16.7% was greater than that observed in any of the other outpatient services.[9]

[6] Aspects of the quantitative analysis of the second year's observations in the cystic fibrosis clinic presented in the subsequent pages, are based upon procedures developed by Robert Ballagh at the Tavistock Institute of Human Relations.

[7] Cf. Appendix B, Table Ib.

[8] Cf. Appendix B, Table XVI, indicating that 65.1% of clinic activities occurred in public areas (waiting room, administration or hall areas) in the second year in orthopedics.

[9] The decline of 16.7% compared with a decrease in family interaction of 1.9% in orthopedic, and of 9.5% in diabetic, while arthritis showed an increase in interaction with families of 20.5%. Cf. Appendix B, Table X, for percentages of staff-family and intra-staff interaction.

Moreover, there was greater involvement with auxiliary and clerical staff. In situations with families present, nursing communication with administrative staff rose from 20.8% to 39.2%.[10] This was largely due to greater nursing entanglement in scheduling of family appointments. The involvement of nursing with clerical matters in cystic fibrosis was accompanied by less reliance on the nurse as source for the resolution of problems.[11]

These trends in the embroilment of the nursing staff in administrative details are confirmed by direct comparison of the data from the various clinics in the new building. In the new cystic fibrosis clinic observed nursing personnel spent 24.1% of their time in administration. This may be compared to figures in the other new clinics: 9.6% in orthopedics, 15.4% in diabetes and 21.5% in arthritis.[12] This emphasis on administration was reflected in the use of the registration desk as a focal point for nursing services. (Thus 25.6% of activities involving the nurse took place in that area. In the orthopedic clinic only 10.3% of nursing services occurred there, while in arthritis and diabetes this location was the site of 10.8% and 16.2% of these activities respectively.[13]

Moreover in time spent in the administrative area as compared to time devoted to areas of primary family contact (the waiting room and the examination rooms) the new cystic fibrosis clinic showed a unique pattern of involvement in administrative red tape. When figures are compared for situations when families were present, the prevalence of prime area usage for family contact (the waiting room and examination room) declined from 95% to 47%.[14] This disruption of the use of prime areas for nursing contact was associated with the discontinuance of the ritual patterns employed by nurses in attempting to deal with the issues of ambivalence and acceptance. It paralleled a rise in administrative family contact in the interstitial areas at the administra-

[10] Cf. Appendix B, Table X, showing an increased clerical involvement of 18.4% in cystic fibrosis, and of 1.3% in diabetes, and decreases of clerical staff contacts of 4.7% in orthopedic and 8.2% in arthritis.

[11] This was reflected in a fall in the nurse's status as an authority referred to for solution of problems, from 63% to 32%. Cf. Appendix B, Table XX, for frequencies on direction of problems to staff and families for resolution.

[12] Cf. Appendix B, Table XVII, for percent of activities by duration in the various outpatient services.

[13] Cf. Appendix B, Table XVI, for percentages on locations-by-duration.

[14] Cf. Appendix B, Table Ib, showing 87% of family first year contact in the waiting room, and 8% in the examination room. The figures for cystic fibrosis activities during the second year were 21.7% in the waiting room, and 25.9% in the examination rooms. Cf. Appendix B, Table XVI.

tion desk and in the corridors from 5% in the old to approximately 17% in the new clinic.

IX-8. Quantitative Evidence of the Decline of Ritual

The mist tent ritual was employed during the first year to cope with longitudinal, life cycle problems. With cystic fibrosis, unlike arthritis, grief inhibited concern with non-medical problems in the home situation.[15] The narrow band of life space considered was indicated by a limited technical emphasis and detailed ritual explanations. This was coupled with a low emphasis on overt emotional problems in the repressed clinic atmosphere. Related to the narrow scope of the ritual approach, a strong emphasis existed on alleviating physical discomfort. This medical approach resulted in an avoidance of issues of the contemporary family life-space.

The pattern of narrow technical disease orientation and longitudinal ritual focus changed noticeably in the new cystic fibrosis clinic. This was reflected in a fall in concern with technical management of the illness, associated with deemphasis of mist tent care, from 53% to 43% during family interaction. Emotional and social problems on the other hand rose from 20% to 34%.[16]

Closely connected with the abandonment of the mist tent rituals was the decline of the nurse as an authority to be sought for in solution of problems. Thus nursing authority fell from 63% to 32%, while physicians as sources for resolution of difficulties showed a rise from 24% to 35%. Families, on the other hand, also showed an increase in authority status from 5% to 12% as bases for appeal for problem solution.[17]

Indication of the greater attention accorded to the immediate difficulties of families was evidenced by staff concern with family transportation, employment difficulties and school problems of children. Attention to this kind of present social difficulties produced a rise in treatment of family-related issues from 14% to 37%.[18] Associated with this greater social (or home-related) approach were gains in family initiation of difficulties from 7% to 21%.[19] These tendencies toward family issues were intimately connected with nursing attempts to provide comfort and sympathy for the children attending the clinic.

[15] Lefton and Rosengren discuss laterality as a system dimension. Cf. M. Lefton and W. R. Rosengren, "Organizations and Clients: Lateral and Longitudinal Dimensions," *American Sociological Review,* **XXXI** (December, 1966), pp. 802-810.

[16] Cf. Appendix B, Table XX, Row 4.

[17] *Ibid.* Row 5.

[18] *Ibid.* Row 2.

[19] *Ibid.* Row 1.

IX-9. Disruption of Ritual and of Support

This greater attention to immediate family social concerns, was counterbalanced by a medical concern with cystic fibrosis as a disease entity. Thus interaction dealing with disease-oriented questions rose from 43% to 58%. At the same time procedures of the hospital in dealing with the illness received scanty interest. Thus hospital treatment recommendations for coping with cystic fibrosis, including especially mist tent care, fell from 43% to 5% of family interaction with the nursing staff.[20]

Nursing efforts to provide comfort to families, and especially to children suffering from cystic fibrosis, was highly understandable in personal terms. However, by concentrating on the overt feelings of families the underlying dynamic of the illness was not confronted.

The discontinuance of the rituals of mist tent care disrupted an important avenue of support for families. The heavy burden of guilt and ambivalence was too great to permit the direct discussion in the clinic of the child's death from the illness. The mist tent explanations by stressing the need for life-long care indirectly raised this issue. By stressing mist tent care, the guilt of parents could be reduced and they could eventually bring themselves and the child to accept his death as a result of the disease.

IX-10. Decline of Ritual Integration of a Family Based Coping Organization

The ecological integration of the clinic through ritual symbolized the bonds of staff and families in coping with the illness. In a personal sense the rituals also were a defense against parental hostility and staff frustration.[21] The ritual prevented these primitive feelings from being expressed. Focused ritual care directed at the issues of guilt and acceptance expressed the solidarity of families and staff as members of a family-oriented life-long coping system.

When the ritual was discontinued the basic issues of guilt and acceptance were no longer appropriately addressed. Ambivalent feelings of fear and frustration surfaced and escape was sought by the staff in unfocused socializing with families or in retreat to administrative areas. This shattered the ecological integration of the clinic as a supportive institution for coping with the issues of guilt and the hereditary death of children.

[20] *Ibid.* Row 2.

[21] Cf. I. Menzies, "A Case Study in the Functioning of Social Systems as a Defense against Anxiety," *Human Relations,* XIII(May, 1960), pp. 95-121.

CHAPTER X

IMPLICATIONS AND CONCLUSION

To families dealing with chronic children's illnesses hospital outpatient services offer an appropriate resource in a social network coping with long-term problems. Through their flexible structure outpatient clinics resonate environmentally in specific stress-related family situations.

This environmental resonance is exemplified by the choice of staff-related areas for treatment focused on problems involving family dependency on medical judgment. Family-related areas promote family autonomy in the management of chronic illnesses.[1]

With the aid of community health networks, families can penetrate the fluid structures of ambulatory care. Negotiations for family health needs are frequently mediated by nurses as "boundary-spanners." The supportive role performance of outpatient nurses with families of chronically ill children is a key focus for the study of family network coping systems.

[1] Cf. Rosengren and De Vault, "The Sociology of Time and Space in an Obstetrical Hospital," in Freidson, ed., *The Hospital in Modern Society,* on the spatially assigned meanings of appropriate and inappropriate behavior in a clinic setting.

X-1. Social Variance and Family Network Support

In facing chronic illnesses of their children families vary within the usual social patterns of family life in their communities; they do not usually deviate from those patterns. The difficulties posed by the disease frequently force families to take extraordinary steps to normalize family life. They may make the child the center of attention, or build much of family social life around health activities related to the illness. In many cases compensatory patterns develop through activities in voluntary health associations.

These associations while valuable as a relief from isolation can also be restrictive to personal and family development. Such constricted patterns may have negative effects on the child emotionally and physically.

In the context of a community social network, the outpatient department comes into focus as a supportive sub-system assisting families in the meaningful social variation of their lives. Outpatient nursing is a boundary spanning discretionary participatory element mediating between the hospital and the home health networks of families.

In this mediating, discretionary role, nursing in its personalized capacity is appropriately equipped for a supportive social variance approach. By virtue of its care function, nursing is free to relate to families in terms of individualized social support rather than in terms of an abstract disease entity. In this discretionary, boundary spanning capacity outpatient nursing care can free the energies of families coping with the long-term stress of chronic illness.[2]

X-2. Community Health Network Factors in Hospital Support

Certain conditions are favorable in the community health network for a supportive hospital response to the social variance needs of chronically ill children. Thus when families are active in voluntary health associations and use such networks for eliciting help from the hospital, the likelihood of hospital support is enhanced. Such networks are apt to be especially effective for this purpose if the disease problems are diffuse and unpredictable. Home health networks can then be used to keep hospital personnel off-balance in dictating the terms of clinic care. Such adversary proceedings are reduced, however, if free and healthy "insider" roles are established by families both in the community and within the hospital structure.

[2] Cf. C. Gersuny and W. R. Rosengren, *The Service Society*, Cambridge, Mass.: The Schenkman Publishing Co., 1973, for discussion of service systems paralleling in certain ways the present analysis of coping systems, but not emphasizing the factor of long term stress.

X-3. Discrepant Conditions for Family Network Support

Receptive forms of hospital support for family coping efforts are especially associated with discrepant institutional patterns. Organizational discrepancies give special range to the improvising capacity of boundary-spannnning personnel.

Thus, in the new arthritis service increased political power combined with weak medical technology in control of the illness gave new supportive opportunities to nursing.[3] The access of nursing to examination rooms enabled families to exploit the potential of a dynamic social network. Familiarity with the clinic along with social support from other families evoked family initiated improvisational processes. Family concern with home-related issues was aired. The intimacy of the examination room was employed by families in raising the issue of acceptance. Nursing support was provided for the anxieties provoked in families attempting to deal with this issue.[4]

Similarly in the diabetic clinic discrepant organizational factors pushed to the fore the supportive role of nursing in family coping networks. In the old diabetic clinic the discretionary powers of nurses as boundary-spanning personnel were minimized by ancillary teaching functions under physician tutelage. With increased discrepancy between the weakness of clinic political power and the adequacy of community resources, nursing discretionary powers were augmented. Alliances were formed with social workers in contacting health services available to families in their home communities.

While the initiative here was more on the side of the hospital, than of the families themselves, a supportive approach to family networks

[3] In contrast with Perrow's interpretation of nursing ability to make independent decisions based on technological factors, discrepancies between technical competence and political power are seen as facilitating such decision-making. Thus high technical competence in a related field (orthopedics) through a "halo" effect (in arthritis) created a surplus of political power which became available for use by nurses. It was the relative strength of surgeons in the structure of decision-making which was the proximate condition for the exercise of power by nurses. Cf. Charles Perrow, "Hospitals: Technology, Structure and Goals," in J. March, *Handbook of Organization,* Chicago: Rand McNally, 1965, pp. 910-971 (especially p. 962).

[4] The leverage exercised by arthritis families over nurses and physicians appeared to be instances of "side-transactions" within Thompson's Type IV "heuristic-optional" model. Nurses appeared anxious to do favors for families in the hope of "completing" the "transaction outcome" of establishing family trust. Such "side-transactions" also enhanced the status of nurses within the clinic. Cf. J. D. Thompson, "Organizations and Output Transactions," *American Journal of Sociology,* LXVIII (November, 1962).

was evident. Increased attention was given to family-related problems not directly connected with the illness. The community approach through social workers, school health departments and visiting nurses indicated an effort to work supportively within the immediate social networks of the families themselves.

X-4. Administrative Support to Families

Certain conditions favor the administrative support functions of discretionary personnel with some families. Thus families facing orthopedic problems which are routine from a medical point of view, feel anxieties about the gravity of the child's condition. These fears are aggravated by the unfamiliarity of crowded conditions such as were experienced in the old orthopedic service. The administrative leadership of nursing in its boundary-spanning discretionary capacity is essential as a mediator for families confronting bureaucratic hospital procedures.[5]

This administrative discretionary function is a case of cultural accretion. The high political power and technical competence of routine orthopedic medicine interposes an impersonal structure. The pleas of families confronting the hospital bureaucracy evoke the mediating role of nursing. This discretionary support for families has no formal recognition within the hospital hierarchy. It also is antithetical to the thrust toward nursing professionalism. Nursing administrative support for families tends to be a cultural accretion without institutional recognition within the health delivery system.[6] It is apt to be swept aside by institutional forces in the process of organizational change.

X-5. Conditions of Ritual Support to Family Networks

Although ritual elements were present in the routine functioning of a large orthopedic service, a more intensified form of ritual marked activities with families dealing with a hereditary fatal children's illness.

[5] Mauksch suggests the possibility of a formalized integrative administrative role for nursing in the context of patient care. Mauksch's discussion parallels the theoretical functionalist analysis of problems of system integration, but within the setting of the hospital structure. Cf. H. Mauksch, "The organizational Context of Nursing Practice," in Fred Davis, ed., *The Nursing Profession: Five Sociological Essays,* New York: John Wiley, 1966, pp. 109-137. Cf. the work of Talcott Parsons on system integration, in *The Social System,* New York: The Free Press of Glencoe, 1951; T. Parsons and R. F. Bales, *Family, Socialization and Interaction Process,* New York: The Free Press of Glencoe, 1955; T. Parsons, *Essays in Sociological Theory,* New York: The Free Press of Glencoe, 1963.

[6] Cf. H. Mauksch, *op. cit.,* for parallel comments on the status of nursing administrative functions.

In the cystic fibrosis clinic, due to absence of an effective medical cure physicians lacked the prestige associated with the surgical departments. Thus surgeons were frequently referred to during nurse-family interaction, but in cystic fibrosis such reference to physicians was very rare.

In the absence of strong medical prestige and of technical effectiveness nursing assumed a ritual pattern of support to families. The ritual mist tent explanations were partly defensive and neutralized the hostility of parents. To the extent that it addressed family responsibility for coping with the illness the ritual dealt with the issues of guilt, acceptance and ambivalence. If families were faithful in their care for the child through mist tent treatment, they reduced their guilt and dealt with the ambivalence of loving the child while seeking escape from the burdens of his illness.

The ritual role of the nurse in the cystic fibrosis clinic was support to the families. This mediation was evident with families who were active in the cystic fibrosis association. They typically interrupted the rituals of the nurse and focused on the actual problems faced in their communities. Nursing support was elicited by families for these home network activities.

Most dramatic were the supportive efforts of the nurse in attempting to encourage families to undertake mist tent care. Such families were frequently not members of an association family network. Stress was evident in interviews with families who had not yet effectively faced their guilt and ambivalence. The strain stemmed in part from the absence of an adequate clinic support structure for the nurse.

X-6. Affective Resources and Ritual Suport

The patterns of affective behavior during activities with cystic fibrosis families indicate specific affective processes. Thus a constant moderate "high" of emotional feeling was maintained both during work and rest periods. This steady "high" patterning violates cultural patterns which dictate that task activities are separated from periods of more intense affective expression. This culturally prescribed patterning was disrupted in the cystic fibrosis clinic as a means of overcoming underlying family despair and depression. This breaking of cultural norms was an instance unique in ego functioning. Here affective resources were drawn upon in a situationally appropriate manner to defend against moods of despair. This steady moderate "high" affectively symbolized the unrelieved stress endured by families coping with the hereditary premature death of their children.[7]

[7] For a related analysis of the functions of ritual, especially in primitive medicine, cf. J. D. Frank, *Persuasion and Healing: A Comparative Study of Psychotherapy*, Baltimore: Johns Hopkins Press, 1961.

X-7. Affective Resources and Improvisational Support

Improvisational patterns in the diabetic and arthritis clinics reveal ego resources in the form of affective channelling. These clinics also departed from the culturally prescribed separation of work activities from intense affective expression. Sensitive feedback response in these clinics was associated with periods of upward movement of feelings during work sequences, and a slightly downward recessive reservoir of emotional activity during relaxed moments. Feelings were actively engaged in a mutual process of social support between families and staff. At the same time feelings, though reduced during periods of rest, were still significantly present.[8]

This social patterning is in line with observations of "natural" groups. Over a life-cycle period groups adopt goals which are collectively important. During activities which are directed toward those goals feelings are more intensively expressed.[9] In situations where activities are of less importance natural groups may relax expression of feelings and maintain a low reservoir (as in the case of the old diabetes clinic).

However, when there is full engagement by a natural group, as with a family, facing long term anxiety, affective channelling may appear. Here anxiety causes a moderate rise in feelings during task sequences. This rise is associated with expectations that the condition can be ameliorated or controlled although it cannot be cured. At the same time feelings are held at a reduced but moderate high during rest as a protection against anxiety. The patterns of affective behavior in dealing with chronic anxiety appear therefore to contrast with the classic analysis of feeling flow typical of "ad hoc" task groups.[10]

The patterns of affective channelling in the diabetes and arthritis clinics, and of affective restraint in cystic fibrosis have interesting implications for the analysis of social support. In all three clinics dominant cultural norms of isolation of feelings from work activities contrasted with the intensified use of feelings during periods of active social support. Exchanges of support between families and staff called

[8] Improvising networks resemble open systems in their ability to maintain active exchange with client environments. Cf. Buckley, *Sociology and Modern Systems Theory,* p. 50.

[9] Improvisational interaction is associated with "wild organization" patterns as defined by Aldrich, while ritualized behavior resembles activities in "domesticated organizations". Cf. Howard Aldrich, "Organizational Boundaries and Inter-organizational Conflict," *Human Relations,* XXIV (August, 1971), pp. 279-293.

[10] Cf. T. Parsons and R. F. Bales, *Family, Socialization and Interaction Process.*

for heightened expression of emotion during work and moderate but significantly evocative behavior during rest.

X-8. Ego Resources, Discrepancy and Institutional Change

The present research suggests that institutional discrepancies are important in liberating the creative powers of discretionary personnel for responding positively to organizational change. Such institutional discrepancies facilitate alliances between families and staff for carrying out supportive activities. These institutional discrepancies are links with the social networks of families. They offer avenues of opportunity to boundary-spanning persons, such as nurses and social workers. They offer entry points into bureaucratized institutions for family coping networks.[11] Such discrepancies offer institutional settings whereby change can be directed in accordance with affective resources made available to the free ego forces of man. In the context of chronic stress problems discrepancies are niches for the development of new institutional types more consonant with the continuity of human life experience.

[11] The trends in the arthritis clinic (and in diabetes) suggest Harrison's analysis of changes "at the level of interpersonal relationships" where "focus is on feelings, attitudes and perceptions." Such "deeper level change" may involve "a radical shift of consultant orientation . . . . accepting a client's felt needs . . . . and working on them at a level where the client can serve as a competent and willing collaborator." Cf. Roger Harrison, "Choosing the Level of Organizational Intervention," *The Journal of Applied Behavioral Science*, VI (April, May, June, 1970), pp. 181-202.

BIBLIOGRAPHY

Agar, John. *Ripping and Running*. New York: Seminar Press, 1973.

Aldrich, Howard. "Organizational Boundaries and Inter-organizational Conflict," *Human Relations*, XXIV (August, 1971), 279-293.

Bales, Robert F. "Adaptive and Integrative Changes as Sources of Strains in Social Systems," *Small Groups: Studies in Social Interaction*. Edited by A. P. Hare, E. F. Borgatta and R. F. Bales. New York: Alfred Knopf, 1965.

Bales, Robert F. *Interaction Process Analysis*. Cambridge: Addison-Wesley Press, 1951.

Balint, M. *The Doctor, His Patient and the Illness*. New York: International Universities Press, 1957.

Bell, Gerald. "Formality versus Flexibility in Complex Organizations," *Organizations and Human Behavior*. Edited by Gerald Bell. Englewood Cliffs, N. J.: Prentice-Hall, 1967, 97-106.

Bell, Norman, and Zucker, Robert. "Family-Hospital Relationships in a State Hospital Setting: A Structural Functional Analysis of the Hospitalization Process," *International Journal of Social Psychiatry*, XV (January, 1964), 73-80.

Berkowitz, N. H, and Bennis, W. G. "Interaction Patterns in Formal Service-Oriented Organizations, *Administrative Science Quarterly*, VI (June, 1961), 25-50.

Blau, Peter M. *Dynamics of Bureaucracy*. Chicago: University of Chicago Press, 1955.

Blau, Peter M. *Exchange and Power in Social Life*. New York: John Wiley and Sons, Inc., 1964.

Bloom, S. W. *The Doctor and His Patient; A Sociological Interpretation*. New York: Free Press, 1965.

Bond, John R., and Vinacke, W. Edgar. "Coalitions in Mixed Sex Triads," *Sociometry*, XXIV (March, 1961), 61-75.

Bott, Elizabeth. *Family and Social Networks: Roles, Norms, and External Relationships in Ordinary Urban Families*. London: Tavistock Publications, 1964.

Brodey, W. M., and Hayden, M. "Intrateam Reactions: Their Relations to the Conflicts of the Family in Treatment," *American Journal of Orthopsychiatry*, XXVII (April, 1957), 349-355.

Bruyn, Severyn T. *The Human Perspective in Sociology: The Methodology of Participant Observation*. Englewood Cliffs, N.J.: Prentice-Hall, 1966.

Buckley, Walter. *Sociology and Modern Systems Theory*. Englewood Cliffs, N.J.: Prentice-Hall, 1967.

Burns, Tom, and Stalker, E. M. *The Management of Innovation*. London: The Tavistock Publications, 1961.

Caplow, Theodore. "A Theory of Coalitions in the Triad," *American Sociological Review*, XXI (August, 1956), 489-493.

Clark, Burton. *Adult Education in Transition: A Study of Institutional Insecurity*. Berkeley: University of California Press, 1968.

Craig, John, and Gross, Edward. "The Forum Theory of Organizational Democracy: Structural Guarantees of Time-Related Variables," *American Sociological Review*, XXXV (February, 1970), 19-33.

Cyert, R., and March, J. *A Behavioral Theory of the Firm*. Englewood Cliffs, N.J.: Prentice-Hall, 1963.

Dayal, Ishmar, and Thomas, John M. "Operation KPE: Developing a New Organization," *Journal of Applied Behavioral Science*, IV (October-December, 1968), 473-506.

De Charms, R. "Affiliation Motivation and Productivity in Small Groups," *Journal of Abnormal and Social Psychology*, LV (1957), 222-226.

Deutsch, Karl W. "Toward a Cybernetic Model of Man and Society," *Modern Systems Research for the Behavioral Scientist: A Sourcebook*. Edited by Walter Buckley. Chicago: Aldine Press, 1968, 387-400.

Dill, William, R. "Environment as an Influence on Managerial Autonomy," *Administrative Science Quarterly*, II (March, 1958), 521-541.

Dumont, Richard G., and Foss, Dennis C. *The American View of Death*. Cambridge, Mass.: Schenkman Publishing Company, 1972.

Duncan, O. D., and Schnore, T. F. "Cultural Behavioral and Ecological Perspectives in the Study of Social Organization," *American Journal of Sociology*, LXV (September, 1959), 132-146.

Erikson, E. H. *Identity and the Life Cycle in Psychological Issues*, Vol. I, No. 1. New York: International Universities Press, 1959.

Etzioni, Amitai (ed.). *The Semi-Professions and Their Organizations: Teachers, Nurses, Social Workers*. New York: Free Press, 1969.

Frank, Jerome David. *Persuasion and Healing, A Comparative Study of Psychotherapy*. Baltimore: Johns Hopkins Press, 1961.

Freidson, Eliot. *Professional Dominance: The Social Structure of Medical Care*. New York: Atherton Press, 1970.

Freidson, Eliot, and Rhea, Buford. "Knowledge and Judgment in Professional Evaluations," *Administrative Science Quarterly*, X (June, 1965), 107-124.

Freidson, Eliot, and Rhea, Buford. "Processes of Control in a Company of Equals," *Social Problems*, XI (Fall, 1963), 119-131.

Freud, Sigmund. "The Instincts and Their Vicissitudes" and "Group Psychology and the Analysis of the Ego," *The Standard Edition of the Complete Psychological Works of S. Freud*. London: Hogarth Press, 1971.

Gamson, W. A. "A Theory of Coalition Formation," *American Sociological Review*, XXVI (June, 1961), 373-382.

Gans, Herbert J. *Urban Villagers*. New York: Free Press of Glencoe, 1962.

Glaser, Barney G., and Strauss, Anselm L. *Awareness of Dying.* Chicago: Aldine Publishing Company, 1965.

Glaser, Barney G., and Strauss, Anselm L. *The Discovery of Grounded Theory: Strategies for Qualitative Research.* Chicago: Aldine Publishing Company, 1967.

Goffman, Erving. *Asylums: Essays on the Social Situation of Mental Patients and Other Inmates.* Chicago: Aldine Publishing Company, 1970.

Goffman, Erving. *Behavior in Public Places; Notes on the Social Organization of Gatherings.* New York: Free Press Paperback, 1968.

Goffman, Erving. *Encounters: Two Studies in the Sociology of Interaction.* Indianapolis: Bobbs-Merrill, 1961.

Goffman, Erving. *The Presentation of Self in Everyday Life,* New York: Doubleday, 1959.

Goode, W. J. "A Theory of Role Strain," *American Sociological Review,* XXV (August, 1960), 483-496.

Gumperz, John, and Hyman, Dill. *New Directions in Sociolinguistics.* New York: Holt, Rinehart and Winston, 1971.

Gurvitch, Georges. *The Spectrum of Social Time,* trans. Myrtle Kovenbaum. Dordrecht: Reidel, 1964.

Hall, A. D., and Fagan, R. E. *Definition of System.* New York: Bell Telephone Laboratories, 1956.

Hare, A. P., Borgatta, E. F., and Bales, R. F. (eds.). *Small Groups: Studies in Social Interaction.* New York: Alfred Knopf, 1965.

Harrison, Roger. "Choosing the Level of Organization Intervention," *The Journal of Applied Behavioral Science,* VI (April, May, June, 1970), 181-202.

Hartman, Heinz. "Notes on the Theory of Sublimation," *Psycho-Analytic Study of the Child,* Vol X. New York: International Universities Press, 1955.

Haug, M. R. and Sussman, M. B. "Professional Autonomy and Revolt of the Client," *Social Problems,* XVII (Fall, 1969), 153-161.

Hawley, A. *Human Ecology: A Theory of Community Structure.* New York: Ronald Press, 1950.

Hughes, E. C. *Men and Their Work.* New York: Free Press of Glencoe, 1958.

Jacques, E. *The Measurement of Responsibility.* London: Tavistock Publications, 1956.

Johnson, M. M., and Martin, H. W. "A Sociological Analysis of the Nursing Role," *In Professionalization.* Edited by Howard M. Vollmer and Donald L. Mills. Englewood Cliffs, N.J., Prentice-Hall, 1966. Reprinted from *American Journal of Nursing,* LVIII (March, 1958).

Kohn, Melvin L. *Class and Conformity: A Study in Values.* Homewood, Ill.: Dorsey Press, 1969.

Kris, Ernst. *Psychoanalytic Explorations in Art.* New York: Schocken Books, 1964.

Leavitt, H., and Mueller, R. "Some Effects of Feedback on Communication," *Small Groups: Studies in Social Interaction.* Edited by A. P. Hare, E. F. Borgatta and R. F. Bales. New York: Alfred Knopf, 1965.

Lefton, M., and Rosengren, W. R. "Organizations and Clients: Lateral and

Longitundinal Dimensions," *American Sociological Review,* XXXI (December, 1966), 802-810.

Lewin, K. "Feedback Problems of Social Diagnosis and Action," *Modern Systems Research for the Behavioral Scientist: A Sourcebook.* Edited by Walter Buckley. Chicago: Aldine Press, 1968.

Lowthrop, Louis C. "The Environment, Bureaucracy and Social Change," *Changing Organizational Behavior.* Edited by A. Bartlett and T. Kayser, Englewood Cliffs, N.J.: Prentice-Hall, Inc., 1973, pp. 19ff.

Lyman, Stanford M., and Scott, Marvin B. "Territoriality: A Neglected Sociological Dimension," *A Sociology of the Absurd.* New York: Appleton-Century-Crofts, 1970.

McClelland, David C. *The Achieving Society.* New York: Collier-Macmillan, 1968.

March, James G. "The Business Firm as a Political Coalition," *Journal of Politics,* XXIV (August, 1962), 662-678.

Mauksch, H. "The Organizational Context of Nursing Practice," *The Nursing Profession: Five Sociological Essays.* Edited by Fred Davis. New York: John Wiley, 1966, 109-137.

Mechanic, David. "Sources of Power of Lower Participants in Complex Organizations," *Administrative Science Quarterly,* VIII (December, 1962), 349-364.

Menzies, I. "A Case Study in the Functioning of Social Systems as a Defense Against Anxiety: A report on a study of the nursing service," *Human Relations,* XIII (May, 1960), 95-121.

Miller, E. Research Monograph. The Tavistock Institute of Human Relations, London, 1972.

Mills, T. M. "The Coalition Pattern in Three Member Groups," *American Sociological Review,* XIX (December, 1954), 657-667.

Mills, T. M. "Power Relations in Three Person Groups," *American Sociological Review,* XVIII (August, 1953), 351-357.

Mills, T. M. *The Sociology of Small Groups.* Englewood Cliffs, N.J.: Prentice-Hall, 1967.

Nathanson, C. "Surveillance and Patient Orientation in a Pediatric Out-Patient Clinic," *Human Organization,* XXX (Fall, 1971), 255-265.

Newcomb, T. M. "An Approach to the Study of Communicative Acts," *Psychological Review,* LX (November, 1953), 393-404.

Parsons, T. *Essays in Sociological Theory.* New York: The Free Press of Glencoe, 1963.

Parsons, T. *The Social System.* New York: Free Press, 1951.

Parsons, T., and Bales, R. F. *Family, Socialization and Interaction Process.* New York: The Free Press of Glencoe, 1955.

Perrow, Charles. "A Framework for the Comparative Analysis of Organizations," *American Sociological Review,* XXXII (April, 1967), 194-208.

Perrow, Charles. "Hospitals: Technology, Structure and Goals," *Handbook of Organization.* Edited by J. March. Chicago: Rand McNally, 1965.

Piaget, Jean. "Social Factors in Moral Development," *Basic Studies in Social Psychology.* Edited by Harold Proshansky and Bernard Seidenberg. New

York: Holt, Rinehart and Winston, 1965. Reprinted from J. Piaget, *The Moral Judgment of the Child,* New York: The Free Press of Glencoe, 1932.

Pill, Roisin. "Space and Social Structure in Two Children's Wards," *Sociological Review,* XV NS (July, 1967), 179-192.

Playa, A. O., Cohen, L. M., and Samora, J. "Communication between Physicians and Patients in Out-Patient Clinics: Social and Cultural Factors," *Millbank Foundation Quarterly,* April, 1968, Vol. 46, No. 2, part 1, 161-213.

Postner, R. S., *et al.* "Process and Outcome in Conjoint Family Therapy," *Family Process,* X (December, 1971), 451-473.

Powell, F. D. "A Concept of Structurated and Destructurated Group Roles: An Initial Empirical Reduction," *Social Science and Medicine,* IV (September, 1970), 321-327.

Psathas, G., and Stryker, S. "Bargaining Behavior and Orientations in Coalition Formation," *Sociometry,* XXVIII (June, 1965), 124-144.

Rapoport, Robert N., with Rhona Rapoport and I. Rosow. *Community as Doctor: New Perspectives on a Therapeutic Community,* London: Tavistock Publications, 1960.

Reiss, Ira L. *The Family System in America.* New York: Holt, Rinehart and Winston, 1971.

Rheingold, Joseph C. *The Mother, Anxiety and Death: the catastrophic death complex.* Boston: Little, Brown, 1967.

Riffenburgh, R. S. "Doctor-patient Relationships in Glaucoma Therapy," *Archives of Opthalmology,* LXXV (July, 1966), 204-206.

Rosengren, W. R., and De Vault, S. "The Sociology of Time and Space in an Obstetrical Hospital," *The Hospital in Modern Society.* Edited by Eliot Freidson. New York: The Free Press, 1963, 266-291.

Roth, J. "Ritual and Magic in the Control of Contagion," *American Sociological Review,* XXII (June, 1956), 310-314.

Roth, J. *Timetables; Structuring the passage of time in hospital treatment and other careers.* Indianapolis: Bobbs-Merril, 1963.

Roth, J. "The Treatment of Tuberculosis as a Bargaining Process," *Human Behavior and Social Process.* Edited by A. Rose. Boston: Houghton Mifflin, 1962, 575-588.

Samuel, Y., and Mannheim, B.H. "A Multidimensional Approach toward a Typology of Bureaucracy," *Administrative Science Quarterly,* XV (March, 1970), 216-228.

Scheff, T. "Negotiating Reality: Notes on Power in the Assessment of Responsibility," *Social Problems,* XVI (Summer, 1968), 3-17.

Schutz, Alfred. *Alfred Schutz on Phenomenology and Social Relations.* Edited by Helmut R. Wagner, Heritage of Sociology Series. Chicago: University of Chicago Press, 1970.

Schutz, Alfred. *Phenomenology of the Social World.* Translated by G. Walsh and F. Lehnert (Studies in Phenomenology and Existential Philosophy Set). Evanston, Ill.: Northwestern University Press, 1967.

Schutz, Alfred. *The Problem of Social Reality,* Vol. I, edited by M. Natanson; *Studies in Social Theory,* Vol. II, edited by A. Broderson; *Studies in Phe-*

nomenological Philosophy, Vol. III, edited by A. Gurvitsch, *Collected Papers.* New York: Humanities Press, Inc., 1962-1966.

Slater, Philip E. *Microcosm.* New York: John Wiley, 1966.

Solomon, Leonard. "Influence of Some Types of Power Relationships and Game Strategies upon the Development of Interpersonal Trust," *Journal of Abnormal and Social Psychology,* LXI (September, 1960), 223-230.

Sommer, Robert. "Studies in Personal Space," *Sociometry,* XXII (September, 1959), 247-260.

Steel, Fred I. *Physical Settings and Organization Development.* Reading, Mass.: Addison-Wesley Publishing Company, 1973.

Strauss, Anselm, *et al.* "The Hospital and its Negotiated Order," *The Hospital in Modern Society.* Edited by Eliot Freidson. New York: Free Press of Glencoe, Inc., 1963.

Strodtbeck. Fred. "The Family as a Three Person Group," *American Sociological Review,* XIX (February, 1954), 23-29.

Sussman, M. B., *et al. The Walking Patient: A Study in Out-Patient Care.* Cleveland: The Press of Western Reserve University, 1967.

Szasz, T., and Hollander, M. "A Contribution to the Philosophy of Medicine." *A.M.A. Archives of Internal Medicine,* Vol. 97, No. 5, (May, 1956), p. 585.

Taylor, C. *In Horizontal Orbit: Hospitals and the Cult of Efficiency.* New York: Holt, Rinehart and Winston, 1970.

Terrien, F., and Mills, D. "The Effect of Changing Size Upon the Structure of Organizations," *American Sociological Review,* XX (February, 1955), 11-13.

Thompson, James D. "Organizations and Output Transactions," *American Journal of Sociology,* LXVIII (November, 1962), 300-324.

Thompson, James D. *Organizations in Action.* New York: McGraw-Hill, 1967.

Thompson, James D., and McEwen, William "Organizational Goals and Environment," *American Sociological Review,* XXIII (February, 1958), 23-31.

Tyler, Stephen. *Cognitive Anthropology.* New York: Holt, Rinehart, 1969.

Voysey, M. "Official Agents and the Legitimation of Suffering," *Sociological Review,* NS XX (November, 1972), 533-551.

Weber, Max. *From Max Weber: Essays in Sociology.* Translated, edited, with an introduction by H. H. Gerth and C. W. Mills. New York: Oxford University Press, 1958.

Wheeler, Stanton. "The Structure of Formally Organized Socialization Settings," *Socialization After Childhood: Two Essays.* By O. Brim and S. Wheeler. New York: John Wiley, 1966.

Whyte, W. F. *Street Corner Society: The Social Structure of an Italian Slum.* Chicago: University of Chicago Press, 1955.

Wilkins, L. T. *Social Deviance.* Englewood Cliffs, N.J.: Prentice-Hall, 1965.

Willis, R. H. "Coalitions in the Tetrad," *Sociometry,* XXV (December, 1962), 358-376.

Zola, Irving. "Problems of Communication, Diagnosis and Patient Care: The Interplay of Patient, Physician and Clinic Organization," *Journal of Medical Education,* XXXVIII (October, 1963), 829-838.

APPENDIX A
METHODOLOGY

A-1. Data Collection for Analysis of Change in Supportive Health Organizations

The data which constitutes the main empirical basis for this analysis of change in institutions providing support to families coping with chronic pediatric illnesses was derived from tape recordings of staff-family and intra-staff interaction in five outpatient services.[1] The formal periods of observation included two periods of two weeks each shortly before and seven months after a move to a larger, modern outpatient building.

The tapes were supplemented by commentary from nurse observers who conducted the recordings. The observers systematically recorded the location, persons present, content of activity and the time of interaction at approximately ten minute intervals. During the first year period comments were obtained from the observers during and immediately after clinic sessions on the content of the recorded data. During the second year period in addition to post-session nursing comments, the observers employed a pre-coded check list form indicating location of the activity, persons entering and leaving the immediate situation, content, and the times of the beginning and end of an in-

[1] Data is also available from a general medical outpatient clinic but is not included in the present report.

teraction.[2] When the clinic nurse, who was being followed, moved to a new location, a new check list form was used indicating a new situation. If a family, nurse or physician left or entered a given location, the new situation was noted.

The recordings and nursing comments were supplemented by interviews with the clinic staff and by home interviews with families.[3] These interviews were of considerable importance in interpreting the meaning of the data gathered during clinic sessions. Since the periods of formal data collection,[4] informal contact has been maintained with the clinics. These contacts suggest a general continuity in the patterns of change associated with the move of the outpatient facilities.[5]

A-2. Initial Data Processing

The clinic tape recordings, observer comments and check list information were transcribed by the research staff. Observer references to unusual emotional expressions such as laughter and crying were also included. Data from the check list was coded and submitted to initial computer analysis focusing on area usage in the diabetic and orthopedic clinics.[6]

A-3. Coding Procedures[7]

The primary level of coding embraced structural and content items which tended to remain constant over longer periods of time. Among these were location of interaction, roles present (family or staff), scope of interactive content (medical, home, or life cycle), initiator and recipient. Identifying data such as clinic and date were also included.[8]

The secondary level embraced process items involving complete thought-sentences, or independent clauses.[9] Second level variables which are of primary interest for the analysis of coping processes include courtship, small talk, feedback, opportunity for feedback, administration and service.[10]

[2] Cf. Check List Form, Appendix, C-1.

[3] Cf. Appendix, C-2, for Home Interview Questionnaire.

[4] 1967 and 1968.

[5] A follow-up study will report on these more recent trends.

[6] Cf. Powell, "A Concept of Structurated and Destructurated Group Roles: An Initial Empirical Reduction," *Social Science and Medicine,* IV (September, 1970).

[7] Developed in collaboration with the Tavistock Institute of Human Relations, London, and The University of Sussex, Falmer, England.

[8] Cf. Code Book, Appendix, C-3, for additional structural and content items.

[9] Consistent with the Bales system of analysis. Cf. R. F. Bales, *Interaction Process Analysis,* Cambridge: Addision-Wesley Press, 1951.

[10] For additional process items cf. Code Book, Appendix, C-3, Cols. 65-79.

A-4. Scaling of a Process Item: Courtship

All process items were coded on five-point rating scales. These scales were established to approximate an equal interval between adjacent points on the scale, consistent with the nature of the interactive data. The first scale point was assigned to absence of behavior being analyzed in accordance with the empirically defined variable.

Thus courtship is a process variable defined as "an emotionally toned attempt by an initiator to elicit interest or action from a recipient."

In accordance with this definition the following rating scale was employed for the variable "courtship":

1. No emotionally toned attempt to elicit interest or action of the other person. (E.g., calling name over P. A. system or behavior involving only one person.)
2. Minimum emotionally toned attempt to elicit interest or action of other person. (E. g., gives information not involving any expectation of response from the other.)
3. Slight emotionally toned atttempt to elicit interest or action of other person. (E. g., seeks information as to convenience of other person regarding routine matter, e.g., time of appointment.)
4. Moderately intense emotionally toned attempt to elicit interest or action of other person. (E. g., tries actively and in friendly manner or using mild warning to induce other to assume responsibility for treatment.)
5. Intense emotional attempt to elicit interest or action of other person. (E. g., uses expression of endearment or coaxing to persuade other of importance of taking responsibility for treatment.)

The scales for the various process items were tested for inter-coder reliability. Average inter-coder reliability was 80% for all process items.[11] The reliability of the items together with the approximately equal interval between scale points was regarded as an appropriate basis for ratio analysis.

The present report based on examination of structural, content, and process items is mainly confined to interaction in which families were present. These items provided the empirical basis for a series of concepts that were developed for interpreting change in the outpatient services viewed as supportive coping organizations.

[11] A more complete discussion of the coding procedures and other aspects of the research methodology is being prepared in collaboration with Margaret Napier.

A-5. Clinic Conceptual Dimensions: Discrete Data

Based on separate and combined uses of the coded items, six concepts were developed for the analysis of the clinics as institutions providing support to families coping with the stress of chronic pediatric illnesses. These concepts are location, initiative, scope, structuring, affectivity and responsiveness.

The clinics are analyzed in terms of two general interactive types derived from specific combinations of four of these conceptual dimensions. Thus *improvising interaction* is associated with the prevalence of family initiative, broad scope, overt affectivity and weak structuring. *Ritual interaction* features relatively intense staff initiatiive, narrow scope, restrained affectivity and rather rigid structuring. *Responsiveness* is positively associated with focused ritual and improvising interaction. Along with these interactive dimensions, health institutions are distinguished ecologically by the organizational *locations* used in providing support to families coping with children's illnesses.

Of the six concepts employed in the analyses, three, *location, initiative* and *scope,* are empirically defined in terms of discrete data; while three are defined by operational use of continuous data: *structuring, responsiveness* and *affectivity.* The first three concepts are based on discrete data in that the data are not conceived in terms of an ordered continuum. Thus "staff initiative" is not ranked in terms of a higher or lower initiating intensity than is "family initiative." In contrast, "structuring" is based on specified combinations of four variables, each ranked within a continuous range of intensity from 1 to 5. (These variables are: courtship, small talk, opportunity for feedback and feedback.)

1. *Location*

   The *location* of typical family-staff contact in a coping institution is conceived as an organizational expression of the issues being supported in families coping with specific children's illnesses.

   Thus outpatient services that stress the use of waiting room areas for family contact use such contact to support family autonomy and acceptance of the illness. Such services insofar as they stress family control of treatment through such waiting room contacts are defined as "family-based."

   Outpatient services that mainly employ examination room contacts with families, use such meetings to support dependency and acceptance of the illness. Such services through supporting dependency and acceptance by means of examination room contact are defined as "staff-based" services.

   Outpatient services stressing interstitial areas (such as the administration desk and corridors) use such contacts to support families' needs to negotiate with the bureaucratic services of the hospital.

Insofar as a clinic such as orthopedics, uses a significant portion of its time for such interstitial area support for such services to families, it may (under certain aspects) be regarded as an "administrative staff-based" system.

Empirically the prominence of support of autonomy and acceptance of the illness is measured by the relative frequency of waiting room contacts with families in a clinic (i.e. family-based contact). Empirically the support of dependency and acceptance of the illness as provided by a clinic is measured by its frequency of examination room contacts with families (i.e. staff-based contact). The degree of support for administrative services to families is empirically measured by the degree of interstitial area contact (i.e. administrative staff-based contact).

2. *Initiative*

The *initiative* of a system is the degree to which staff or families assume control over the interaction. The concept "initiative" is empirically defined by the percentage of staff-family interaction that is initiated by families compared with the percent initiated by the staff. Family initiative is associated with improvisation and staff initiative is an element of ritual interactive patterns. (Cf. Table II for percent overall family initiative.)

As shown in Table II, Appendix B, below, comparisons have been made for percentages and frequencies of family *initiative* both by *location* and by *scope*. The combined comparisons of these discrete conceptualized variables are discussed in the main body of the present report. Further comparisons involving both discrete and continuous conceptual variables will be contained in subsequent analyses of the data.

3. *Scope*

Scope is the degree of narrowness or breadth that characterizes the content of interaction (cf. "laterality" and "longitudinality" as discussed by Lefton and Rosengren, *op.cit.).* Empirically the percentage of staff or family initiative focused in terms of *medical* (narrow scope), *home* or *life-cycle* (broad scope) issues determines the scope of a given clinic's interaction.[12] *Medical* scope is associated with ritual patterns, while *home* and *life-cycle* scope are associated with improvisation. (Cf. Tables Ia and Ib, Appendix B.)

A-6. Clinic Conceptual Dimensions Based on Continuous Data

1. *Structuring*

[12] Scope is also indicated by the stability of a given content of communication over time as indicated by sequential or lagged correlation analysis. Cf. Table III, Appendix B.

Structuring is related to *initiative* insofar as both concepts deal with the control over family-staff interaction. Initiative is concerned with the quantity of such family or staff control. Structuring focuses on the qualitative distribution of such control.

In the present context, *structuring* is defined by the degree to which individual clinic interaction accords with patterns of role assumption characteristic of overall outpatient behavior in the health delivery network. This overall role assumption pattern shows families dominant in initiating small talk and feedback, with staff initiative prevalent in courtship and opportunity for feedback.

Structuring is empirically measured by differences in lagged correlations for family and staff initiative on these four variables in the assigned role direction. The lagged correlations were derived from an act-by-act or sequential analysis of the four variables measuring the relation of the intensity of each variable to staff or family initiation. Two cumulative four-step matrices were thus developed. Differences in staff and family correlations were measured at the first step in each matrix. (Cf. Tables IV and V, Appendix B.)

Structuring is associated positively with ritual interaction and negatively with improvisation.

2. *Responsiveness*

   Responsiveness is the degree of sensitivity in a communication network and is empirically defined by the unique variance as derived from the lagged regression analysis of feedback (at lag 1) as related to opportunity for feedback. Focused ritual and improvisation are positively associated with responsiveness. (Cf. Table VI, Appendix B.)

3. *Affectivity*

   Affectivity denotes the manner in which feelings are put forth or withheld during work and non-work situations. In the present research the concept is operationally defined in terms of an analysis of cross-tabulations of courtship and small talk; courtship and opportunity for feedback; and courtship and service.

   The cross-tabulations were condensed by a weighting procedure which assigned high and low joint levels both to affective and to task variables.[13] Values of 1 and 2 were assigned low intensity, while 3, 4 and 5 were given high intensity ratings. The weighting procedure involved multiplication of the frequencies in the cross-tabulations by the intensities found in a given cell.[14]

[13] Cf. Tables XXI to XXVI, Appendix B, for cross-tabulations from the diabetic clinic.

[14] Column I was dropped from the analysis since a predominance of unob-

The result of this manipulation was a four-fold distribution of the data: high intensity feelings with low work activity; high intensity feelings with high work activity; low intensity feelings with low work activity; and low intensity feelings with high work activity.

The high feeling-low work activity total was divided by the sum of the two low feeling categories. This yielded a Reservoir Ratio representing the prevalence of high intensity feelings not put to work relative to all low level feelings.

The high feeling-high work activity total was divided by the sum of low feeling values. The result was an Expression Ratio representing the strength of high intensity feelings put to work relative to unexpressed feelings.

Based on the Reservoir and Expression Ratios, various affective patterns are derived. Thus a high Expression Ratio and relatively low Reservoir Ratio produce Affective Diffusion. (Cf. Table VII, Appendix B—Diabetic Clinic, 1st Year—Col. 4: Expression Ratio = 3.620; Col. 3: Reservoir Ratio = 0.823.)

A moderately high Expression Ratio with a somewhat lower Reservoir Ratio yields a pattern of Affective Channelling. (Cf. Appendix B, Table VII—Arthritis, 2nd Year—Col. 4: Expression Ratio = 1.777; Col. 3: Reservoir Ratio = 0.795.)

Nearly equal Expression and Reservoir Ratios with perhaps some positive Expression bias produce Affective Restraint. (Cf. Appendix B, Table VII—Cystic Fibrosis, 1st Year—Col. 4: Expression Ratio = 0.872; Col. 3: Reservoir Ratio = 0.828:

A slight excess of the Reservoir over the Expression Ratio indicates a pattern of Affective Suppression. (Cf. Appendix B, Table VII—Scoleosis, 1st Year—Col. 4: Expression Ratio = 0.581; Col. 3: Reservoir Ratio = 0.959.)

A moderate to high dominance of the Reservoir Ratio over the Expression Ratio reveals a model of Affective Isolation. (Cf. Appendix B, Table VII—Orthopedic, 1st Year—Col. 4: Expression Ratio = 0.456; Col. 3: Reservoir Ratio = 1.081.)

These patterns are each cognate with ritual or improvisation: isolated, suppressed and restrained feelings mark ritualized interaction; channelling and diffusion are associated with improvisational activity.

served behavior occurred in the instrumental categories. Row 1 was retained because affective behavior was more normally distributed, and appeared more meaningful as an indication of failure to express feeling. The variable "courtship" was assigned a task role relative to "small talk", but was viewed as affect relative to "opportunity for feedback" and "service".

APPENDIX B
TABLES

Table Ia

PERCENTAGE SCOPE BY CLINIC (Family-Staff Interaction)

	Arthritis				Diabetic				Orthopedic				Cystic Fibrosis	
Year	1st		2nd		1st		2nd		1st		2nd		1st	
	M	H/L	M	H/L	M	H/L	M	H/L	M	H/L	M	H/L	M	H/L
	45	55	49	51	87	13	69	31	67	33	62	38	89	11

Table Ib

PERCENT SCOPE BY LOCATION (Family-Staff Interaction)

	Arthritis						Diabetic						Orthopedic						Cystic Fibrosis		
Year	1st			2nd			1st			2nd			1st			2nd			1st		
	M	H	L	M	H	L	M	H	L	M	H	L	M	H	L	M	H	L	M	H	L
WR		2					48	7	2	32	21	3	4	2		3			76	10	1
AD	1			6						3			1						5		
CORR				7	3	6	6	2		5			4	1		2					
ER	44	36	17	36	30	12	33	2		22	5	2	53	18	12	52	25	12	8		
CR													3								
OUT										7			2					6			
OTHER																					

Key:

Scope
- M = Medical
- H = Home
- L = Life cycle

Location
- WR = Waiting Room
- AD = Administrative Desk
- CORR = Corridor
- ER = Examination Room
- CR = Cast Room

Table II

FREQUENCY OF FAMILY-STAFF INITIATIONS (f) AND PERCENT (%) OF INTERACTIONS INITIATED BY FAMILIES AT A SPECIFIC LOCATION AND SCOPE

Location	Arthritis Clinic				Diabetic Clinic				Orthopedic Clinic				Cystic Fibrosis Clinic	
	1st Yr.		2nd Yr.		1st Yr.		2nd Yr.		1st Yr.		2nd Yr.		1st Yr.	
Scope	f	%	f	%	f	%	f	%	f	%	f	%	f	%
Waiting Rm.														
Medical					893	31.5%	710	24.6%	129	28.7%	42	40.5%	1756	34.4%
Home					144	49.3%	342	36.0%	41	36.6%	3	33.3%	238	54.2%
Life					34	08.8%	49	16.3%					17	35.3%
Admin. Desk														
Medical			80	00.0%			60	15.0%	36	16.7%	9	0.00	111	36.0%
Home							24	37.5%					29	75.9%
Life							6	33.3%						
Corridor														
Medical			110	38.2%	108	25.0%	101	25.7%	126	31.7%	30	16.7%		
Home			65	50.8%	44	54.5%	23	47.8%	36	47.2%				
Life			104	40.4%							3	33.3%		
Exam. Rm.														
Medical	183	31.7%	631	43.1%	647	19.3%	301	40.5%	1546	34.0%	744	31.2%	179	22.9%
Home	155	68.4%	529	55.8%	45	24.4%	65	61.5%	553	50.5%	355	51.3%		
Life	82	32.9%	216	39.4%			43	51.2%	381	38.8%	171	43.1%		

Cast Rm. Medical					93 30.1%		
Outside Medical					47 23.4%		
Other Medical						46 19.6%	
Home				117 06.8%		15 40.0%	

	Arthritis Clinic		Diabetic Clinic		Orthopedic Clinic		Cystic Fibrosis Clinic
	1st Yr.	2nd Yr.	1st Yr.	2nd Yr.	1st Yr.	2nd Yr.	1st Yr.
Total staff-family interaction	F=420	F=1735	F=1915	F=1841	F=2988	F=1421	F=2330
% of total interaction initiated by family	44.3%	44.2%	28.5%	30.1%	36.7%	37.1%	36.4%

Percentages (%) given refer to initiation by families while frequencies (f) refer to all interactions initiated by families *and* staff. Thus 893 interactions were initiated by staff and families at medical scope in the waiting room in the diabetic clinic during the first year. Of these total interactions, 31.5% were initiated by families and 68.5% were initiated by staff. Thus percentages presented in the table do not add to 100%.

Table III

STABILITY OF INTERACTION OVER TIME BY SCOPE (as measured by lagged Correlations*)

Clinic & Year	Lag 1 Scope Medical	Lag 1 Scope Home	Lag 1 Scope Life	Lag 2 Scope Medical	Lag 2 Scope Home	Lag 2 Scope Life	Lag 3 Scope Medical	Lag 3 Scope Home	Lag 3 Scope Life
Arthritis									
1st	.881	.896	.872	.771	.802	.758	.670	.708	.658
2nd	.884	.901	.907	.781	.811	.834	.673	.729	.768
Diabetic									
1st	.657	.751	.414	.498	.633	.282	.388	.536	.171
2nd	.691	.706	.551	.497	.518	.416	.389	.398	.236
Orthopedic									
1st	.742	.775	.484	.564	.617	.139	.389	.505	.033
2nd	.765	.719	.846	.553	.433	.731	.388	.288	.616
Cysticfibrosis									
1st	.671	.736	.725	.460	.537	.633	.319	.408	.547

*Cf. Methodology, Appendix A, Section A-6-1, for discussion of the use of lagged correlations in the analysis of interaction over time.

Table IV

DATA ON INTERACTIVE STRUCTURING AT MEDICAL SCOPE*

ARTHRITIS

1st Yr.: N = 199; Overall total expected positive & negative correlations = 1.296
2nd Yr.: N = 749; Overall total expected positive & negative correlations = 0.782

	Courtship	Exp. Corr. Total	Small Talk	Exp. Corr. Total	Feedback	Exp. Corr. Total	Opp. for Feedback	Exp. Corr. Total
1st year								
Fam. Init.	-0.278		0.223		0.300		-0.196	
		.380		.257		.481		.178
Staff Init.	0.102		-0.034		-0.181		-0.018	
2nd year								
Fam. Init	-0.086		0.146		0.089		0.050	
		.161		.358		.159		-.104
Staff Init.	0.075		-0.212		-0.070		-0.054	

ORTHOPEDIC

1st Yr.: N = 1987; Overall total expected positive & negative correlations = 0.911
2nd Yr.: N = 1680; Overall total expected positive & negative correlations = 0.944

	Court-ship	Exp. Corr. Total	Small Talk	Exp. Corr. Total	Feed-back	Exp. Corr. Total	Opp. for Feedback	Exp. Corr. Total
1st year								
Fam. Init.	-0.190		-0.029		0.217		-0.154	
		.348		-.099		.396		.266
Staff Init.	0.158		0.070		-0.179		0.112	
2nd year								
Fam. Init.	-0.169		-0.031		0.282		-0.154	
		.351		-.149		.372		.370
Staff Init.	0.182		0.113		-0.190		0.216	

CYSTIC FIBROSIS

1st Yr.: N = 3050; Overall total expected positive & negative correlations = 1.541

	Court-ship	Exp. Corr. Total	Small Talk	Exp. Corr. Total	Feed-back	Exp. Corr. Total	Opp. for Feedback	Exp. Corr. Total
1st year								
Fam. Init.	-0.375		-0.130		0.340		-0.190	
		.768		-.276		.671		.378
Staff Init.	0.393		0.146		-0.331		0.188	

SCOLEOSIS

1st Yr.: N = 1142; Overall total expected positive & negative correlations = 1.178

	Court-ship	Exp. Corr. Total	Small Talk	Exp. Corr. Total	Feed-back	Exp. Corr. Total	Opp. for Feedback	Exp. Corr. Total
1st year								
Fam. Init.	-0.241		-0.047		0.263		-0.134	.265
		.503		-.115		.524		
Staff Init.	0.262		0.068		-0.261		0.131	

*As measured by total positive and negative correlations in expected directions.
Cf. Methodology, Appendix A, Sect. A-6-1, for empirical definition of structuring.
Expected directions of correlations: Family positive on small talk and feedback.
Staff positive on courtship and opportunity feedback.

Table V

DATA ON INTERACTIVE STRUCTURING AT LIFE CYCLE, HOME AND MEDICAL SCOPES* DIABETES CLINIC

Life Cycle Scope

1st Yr.: N = 47; Overall total expected positive & negative correlations = 1.362
2nd Yr.: N = 102; Overall total expected positive & negative correlations = 2.024

	Court-ship	Exp. Corr. Total	Small Talk	Exp. Corr. Total	Feed-back	Exp. Corr. Total	Opp. for Feedback	Exp. Corr. Total
1st year								
Fam. Init.	-0.189		-0.037		0.385		-0.114	
		.457		-.043		.688		.260
Staff Init.	0.268		0.006		-0.303		0.146	
2nd year								
Fam. Init.	-0.389		0.060		0.314		-0.226	
		.733		.157		.708		.426
Staff Init.	0.344		-0.097		-0.394		0.200	

Home Scope

1st Yr.: N = 233; Overall total expected positive & negative correlations = 2.075
2nd Yr.: N = 467; Overall total expected positive & negative correlations = 1.417

	Court-ship	Exp. Corr. Total	Small Talk	Exp. Corr. Total	Feed-back	Exp. Corr. Total	Opp. for Feedback	Exp. Corr. Total
1st year								
Fam. Init.	-0.184		0.102		0.353		-0.337	
		.418		.221		.690		.736
Staff Init.	0.234		-0.119		-0.337		0.399	
2nd year								
Fam. Init.	-0.298		0.024		0.224		-0.167	
		.573		.075		.434		.335
Staff Init.	0.275		-0.051		-0.210		0.168	

Medical Scope

1st Yr.: N = 1648; Overall total expected positive & negative correlations = 1.603
2nd Yr.: N = 1276; Overall total expected positive & negative correlations = 1.388

	Court-ship	Exp. Corr. Total	Small Talk	Exp. Corr. Total	Feed-back	Exp. Corr. Total	Opp. for Feedback	Exp. Corr. Total
1st year								
Fam. Init.	-0.187		0.051		0.430		-0.238	
		.368		-.003		.760		.478
Staff Init.	0.181		0.054		-0.330		0.240	
2nd year								
Fam. Init.	-0.399		-0.081		0.269		-0.099	
		.782		-.124		.543		.187
Staff = Init.	0.383		0.043		0.274		0.088	

*As measured by total positive and negative correlations in expected directions.
Cf. Methodology, Appendix A, Sect. A-6-1, for discussion of structuring.
Expected directions of correlations: Staff positive on courtship and opportunity for feedback. Family positive on small talk and feedback.

Table VI

DATA ON FEEDBACK RESPONSIVENESS (INDICATED BY UNIQUE VARIANCE AT LAG 1 OF FEEDBACK AS RELATED TO IMMEDIATELY PRIOR OPPORTUNITY FOR FEEDBACK)

Year	Family Initiation		Staff Initiation
		Arthritis	
1st	06.7%		35.3%
2nd	21.0%		37.8%
		Cystic Fibrosis	
1st	25.7%		34.0%
2nd	——		——
		Diabetic	
1st	13.8%		18.5%
2nd	27.7%		24.4%
		Orthopedic	
1st	26.2%		24.2%
2nd	09.1%		25.7%
		Scoleosis	
1st	32.4%		29.6%

(Derived from lagged regression analysis.)

Table VII

COMPONENTS OF AFFECTIVITY MEASUREMENT

Col. 1	2	3	4	5	6
Clinic	Year	Reservoir Ratio (mean for 3 ratios *re* reserved affect÷by low affect)	Expression Ratio (mean for 3 ratios *re* expressed affect÷by low affect)	Difference of Affect Ratios (Col. 4 -Col. 3) (+) = ER > RR (-) = ER < RR	Mean of Affect Ratios (Col. 4 +Col. 3) ÷2
Arthritis	1st	0.782	1.001	+0.219	0.892
Arthritis	2nd	0.795	1.777	+0.982	1.286
Diabetic	1st	0.823	3.620	+2.797	2.221
Diabetic	2nd	0.508	1.001	+0.493	0.755
Orthopedic	1st	1.081	0.456	-0.625	0.769
Orthopedic	2nd	0.379	0.588	+0.209	0.486
Cystic Fibrosis	1st	0.828	0.872	+0.044	0.848
Scoleosis	1st	0.959	0.581	-0.374	0.770

Table VIII

AFFECTIVE RATIO COMPARISONS

Based on Cross-Tabulation Analysis of Arthritis and Diabetic Clinics

Col. 1	2	3	4	5	6	7
Clinic	Year	Categories Compared	Reservoir Ratio	Expression Ratio	Sum of Affective Ratios	Diff. in Affective Ratios
Arthritis	1st	Small Talk x Courtship	2.233	1.594	3.827	-0.639
Arthritis	2nd	Small Talk x Courtship	2.044	2.351	4.395	+0.327
Arthritis	1st	Courtship x Opp. Feed.	0.033	0.704	0.737	+0.671
Arthritis	2nd	Courtship x Opp. Feed.	0.074	2.328	2.402	+2.254
Arthritis	1st	Courtship x Service	0.079	0.705	0.784	+0.626
Arthritis	2nd	Courtship x Service	0.268	0.651	0.919	+0.383
Arthritis	1st	Total: 3 Comparisons	2.345	3.003	5.348	+0.658
Arthritis	1st	Average: 3 Comparisons	0.782	1.001	1.783	+0.219
Arthritis	2nd	Total: 3 Comparisons	2.386	5.330	7.716	+2.944
Arthritis	2nd	Average: 3 Comparisons	0.795	1.777	2.572	+0.982
Diabetic	1st	Small Talk x Courtship	0.550	4.394	4.944	+3.844
Diabetic	2nd	Small Talk x Courtship	1.195	1.244	2.439	-0.049
Diabetic	1st	Courtship x Opp. Feed.	0.048	3.691	3.739	+3.643
Diabetic	2nd	Courtship x Opp. Feed.	0.034	0.913	0.947	+0.879
Diabetic	1st	Courtship x Service	1.871	2.774	4.645	+0.903
Diabetic	2nd	Courtship x Service	0.296	0.845	1.141	+0.549
Diabetic	1st	Total: 3 Comparisons	2.469	10.859	13.032	+8.390
Diabetic	1st	Average: 3 Comparisons	0.823	3.620	4.443	+2.797
Diabetic	2nd	Total: 3 Comparisons	1.525	3.002	4.527	+1.477
Diabetic	2nd	Average: 3 Comparisons	0.508	1.001	1.508	+0.493

Table IX

AFFECTIVE RATIO COMPARISONS

Based on Cross-Tabs: Orthopedics, Cystic Fibrosis, Scoleosis Clinics

Col. 1	2	3	4	5	6	7
Clinic	Year	Categories Compared	Reservoir Ratio	Expression Ratio	Sum of Affective Ratios	Diff. in Affective Ratios
Orthoped.	1st	Small Talk x Courtship	3.188	0.938	4.076	-2.250
Orthoped.	2nd	Small Talk x Courtship	0.914	0.651	1.565	-0.263
Orthoped.	1st	Courtship x Opp. Feed.	0.014	0.223	0.237	+0.209
Orthoped.	2nd	Courtship x Opp. Feed.	0.061	0.697	0.758	+0.636
Orthoped.	1st	Courtship x Service	0.042	0.208	0.250	+0.166
Orthoped.	2nd	Courtship x Service	0.162	0.417	0.579	+0.255
Orthoped.	1st	Total: 3 Comparisons	3.244	1.369	4.613	-1.875
Orthoped.	1st	Average: 3 Comparisons	1.081	0.456	1.537	-0.625
Orthoped.	2nd	Total: 3 Comparisons	1.137	1.765	2.902	+0.628
Orthoped.	2nd	Average: 3 Comparisons	0.379	0.588	0.983	+0.209
Cystic F.	1st	Small Talk x Courtship	2.271	1.731	4.002	-0.540
Cystic F.	1st	Courtship x Opp. Feed.	0.082	0.670	0.752	+0.568
Cystic F.	1st	Courtship x Service	0.131	0.216	0.347	+0.085
Cystic F.	1st	Total: 3 Comparisons	2.484	2.617	5.101	+0.133
Cystic F.	1st	Average: 3 Comparisons	0.828	0.872	1.701	+0.044
Scoleosis	1st	Small Talk x Courtship	2.688	1.148	3.836	-1.540
Scoleosis	1st	Courtship x Opp. Feed.	0.011	0.411	0.422	+0.400
Scoleosis	1st	Courtship x Service	0.177	0.184	0.361	+0.007
Scoleosis	1st	Total: 3 Comparisons	2.876	1.743	4.619	-1.133
Scoleosis	1st	Average: 3 Comparisons	0.959	0.581	1.540	-0.374

Table X

PERCENT INTERACTION WITH STAFF, PHYSICIANS AND FAMILY
(based on line count of transcripts)

N = Number of lines

CLINIC	STAFF	PHYSI-CIANS	FAMILY	STAFF	PHYSI-CIANS	FAMILY
Orthopedic	1st year: N=16,995			2nd year: N=4308		
Percent each year	44.8%	11.6%	43.6%	40.1%	18.2%	41.7%
Diabetic	1st year: N=3160			2nd year: N=3095		
Percent each year	15.5%	19.9%	64.6%	16.8%	28.1%	55.1%
Arthritis	1st year: N=649			2nd year: N=1457		
Percent each year	25.0%	17.6%	57.5%	16.8%	5.2%	78.0%
Cystic Fibrosis	1st year: N=7199			2nd year: N=7101		
Percent each year	20.8%	17.2%	62.0%	39.2%	17.0%	43.8%
Scoleosis	1st year: N=2210					
Percent each year	14.8%	24.8%	60.4%			

Table XI

ARTHRITIS
Frequencies and Percentages
FAMILY-NURSE INTERACTION

	1st year: Total Word Frequency = 2320				2nd year: Total Word Frequency = 7429			
	Nurse to Parents	Parents to Nurse	Nurse to Patient	Patient to Nurse	Nurse to Parents	Parents to Nurse	Nurse to Patient	Patient to Nurse
Freq.	953	1193	161	13	3080	3278	901	13
Percent of Total	41.1%	51.4%	6.9%	0.6%	41.5%	44.1%	12.1%	2.3%

Based on 9749
Family-Nurse Interaction Words

Table XII

DIABETIC
Frequencies and Percentages
FAMILY-NURSE INTERACTION
(based on line count)

	1st year: Total Frequency = 1522				2nd year: Total Frequency = 1410			
	Nurse to Parents 1	Parents to Nurse 2	Nurse to Patient 3	Patient to Nurse 4	Nurse to Parents 1	Parents to Nurse 2	Nurse to Patient 3	Patient to Nurse 4
Freq.	388	350	621	163	558	334	382	136
Percent of Total	25.5%	23.0%	40.8%	10.7%	39.6%	23.7%	27.1%	9.6%

Based on 17,592
Family-Nurse Interaction Words

Table XIII

ORTHOPEDIC
Frequencies and Percentages
FAMILY-NURSE INTERACTION
(based on line count)

	1st year: Total Frequency = 4366				2nd year: Total Frequency = 1190			
	Nurse to Parents	Parents to Nurse	Nurse to Patient	Patient to Nurse	Nurse to Parents	Parents to Nurse	Nurse to Patient	Patient to Nurse
Freq.	2189	1462	545	170	475	379	251	85
Percent of Total	50.1%	33.5%	12.5%	3.9%	39.9%	31.8%	21.1%	7.1%

Based on 33,236
Family-Nurse Interaction Words

Table XIV

3RD PERSON PRONOUN USAGE REFERRING TO PHYSICIANS AND TO PATIENTS

Year	Clinic (or Type of Clinic Sequence)	Total Lines	3rd Person Reference to Physician		3rd Person Reference to Patient		Ratio of 3rd Person reference to Patient vs. Reference to Physician Col. 5 ÷ by Col. 3
			N	R	N	R	
	1	2	3	4	5	6	7
Both	Orthopedic	8978	378	23.75	2579	3.48	6.82
1st		6949	329	21.12	2068	3.36	6.29
2nd		2029	49	41.41	511	3.97	10.43
Both	Diabetic	3689	125	29.51	947	3.90	7.58
1st		1906	48	39.71	502	3.80	10.46
2nd		1783	77	23.16	445	4.01	5.81
1st	Cystic Fibrosis (Mist Tent Sequences)	1497	0	00	132	11.34	132.00
1st	Cystic Fibrosis (Other Sequences)	2335	10	233.50	574	4.06	57.40
1st	Scoleosis	707	68	10.39	146	4.84	2.15
Both	Arthritis	2012	112	17.96	859	2.34	7.67
1st		597	19	31.42	255	2.34	13.42
2nd		1415	93	15.22	604	2.34	6.49
	Total	19218	693		5237		
	Mean			27.73		3.67	13.98

N = Frequency of Specified Pronoun Use

R = Total lines (as shown in Col. 2) divided by N.

Table XV

PRONOUN USES BY CLINIC FAMILY MEMBERS

Year	Clinic (or Type of Clinic Sequence)	Total Lines	1st Person Singular Initiations *By Patient Mother* N	R	1st Person Plural Initiations *By Patient Mother* N	R
	1	2	3	4	5	6
Both	Orthopedic	8978	626	14.34	76	118.13
1st		6949	459	15.14	61	113.92
2nd		2029	167	12.15	15	135.27
Both	Diabetic	3689	183	20.16	50	73.78
1st		1906	136	14.01	43	44.33
2nd		1783	47	37.94	7	254.71
1st	Cystic Fibrosis (Mist tent Sequences)	1497	163	9.18	89	16.82
					} 129	} 29.71
1st	Cystic Fibrosis (other Sequences)	2335	182	12.83	40	58.38
Both	Scoleosis	707	109	6.49	20	35.35
Both	Arthritis	2012	194	10.37	38	52.95
Total		19218	1457		313	
Mean				13.19		61.40

N = No. of pronouns by category.
R = No. of lines shown in Col. 2 divided by N.

Table XVI

LOCATION BY DURATION
(Percent: Based on Checklist data for second year)

	W.R.	A.D.	Hall	N.S.	R.R.	Ex R.	C.R.	Out & Other
Orthopedic	2.2	10.3	12.0	9.6	8.1	31.2	8.7	17.8
Arthritis	0	10.8	29.0	6.8	3.4	50.0		
Diabetic	48.0	16.2	11.8	4.3	5.2	11.8		2.6
Cystic Fibrosis	21.1	25.6	18.4	2.3	2.7	25.9		4.0

Key to Locations:

W.R. = Waiting Room
A.D. = Administration Desk
Hall = Hallway or Corridor
R.R. = Residents' Room
Ex.R. = Examination Room
C.R. = Cast Room
Out = Outside the clinic
Other or unidentified locations

Table XVII

PERCENT ACTIVITY BY DURATION
(Based on Checklist data for second year)

	Teaching	Information	Service	Administration	Social
Orthopedic	17.3	17.4	30.3	9.6	25.3
Arthritis	28.8	25.4	19.2	21.5	5.1
Diabetic	58.2	17.9	4.1	15.4	4.4
Cystic Fibrosis	20.3	32.2	18.1	24.1	5.4

Table XVIII

MEANS FOR PROCESS VARIABLES*
ARTHRITIS AND ORTHOPEDIC CLINICS

	ARTHRITIS							
	1st Year				2nd Year			
Variables	Family Initia-tion		ETA	Staff Initia-tion	Family Initia-tion		ETA	Staff Initia-tion
Courtship	1.804	x	03.5%	2.140	2.112	x	01.6%	2.357
Small Talk	2.970	x	10.3%	2.298	3.206	x	01.7%	2.951
Feedback	1.658	x	11.2%	1.038	1.245	x	01.6%	1.090
Opp. Feedback	1.226	x	06.7%	1.860	1.296	x	00.2%	1.389
Med. Information	1.407	x	00.8%	1.553	1.242	x	00.8%	1.362
Service	1.000	x	12.0%	1.532	1.057	x	06.1%	1.406
Administration	1.000	x	01.6%	1.072	1.000	x	01.4%	1.011

	ORTHOPEDIC							
	1st Year				2nd Year			
Variables	Family Initia-tion		ETA	Staff Initia-tion	Family Initia-tion		ETA	Staff Initia-tion
Courtship	1.575	x	05.4%	1.933	1.606	x	03.8%	1.961
Small Talk	2.798	x	00.1%	2.848	2.622	x	00.1%	2.564
Feedback	1.395	x	05.7%	1.079	1.335	x	08.1%	1.029
Opp. Feedback	1.302	x	04.5%	1.869	1.153	x	04.6%	1.626
Med. Information	1.192	x	00.4%	1.271	1.213	x	03.2%	1.472
Service	1.031	x	28.0%	2.069	1.036	x	17.4%	1.720
Administration	1.012	x	03.0%	1.189	1.006	x	00.4%	1.028

* Based on Five Point Scales.

Table XIX

MEANS FOR PROCESS VARIABLES*
DATA FROM DIABETES, CYSTIC-FIBROSIS, SCOLEOSIS

	DIABETES							
	1st Year				2nd Year			
Variables	Family Initiation		ETA	Staff Initiation	Family Initiation		ETA	Staff Initiation
Courtship	2.798	x	03.3%	3.300	1.454	x	14.4%	2.287
Small Talk	3.171	x	00.7%	2.957	2.600	x	00.1%	2.651
Feedback	1.881	x	18.0%	1.067	1.546	x	07.3%	1.119
Opp. Feedback	1.301	x	05.7%	2.044	1.397	x	01.6%	1.742
Med. Information	1.572	x	01.2%	1.858	1.366	x	03.4%	1.728
Service	1.083	x	00.7%	1.194	1.020	x	03.9%	1.297
Administration	1.002	x	00.9%	1.069	1.011	x	00.3%	1.036

	CYSTIC FIBROSIS				SCOLEOSIS			
	1st Year				1st Year			
Variables	Family Initiation		ETA	Staff Initiation	Family Initiation		ETA	Staff Initiation
Courtship	1.410	x	16.6%	2.151	1.514	x	06.6%	1.988
Small Talk	2.710	x	00.6%	2.806	2.741	x	00.0%	2.752
Feedback	1.569	x	11.9%	1.091	1.426	x	08.2%	1.060
Opp. Feedback	1.309	x	05.2%	1.966	1.245	x	03.3%	1.706
Med. Information	1.483	x	03.2%	1.804	1.370	x	00.3%	1.466
Service	1.023	x	10.9%	1.597	1.006	x	20.7%	1.810
Administration	1.000	x	00.4%	1.018	1.000	x	02.3%	1.121

* Based on Five Point Scales.

Table XX

ANALYSIS OF PROBLEM SOLVING PROCESS CYSTIC FIBROSIS CLINIC (N.B. all figures are percentages, with raw scores in parenthesis)

	% Problem Units		1st Year	2nd Year
Row 1	*Raised by:*	Nurse	64 (95)	74 (44)
		Doctor	14 (21)	
		Family	7 (10)	21 (12)
		Hospital	9 (14)	
		Other	5 (8)	5 (3)
Row 2	*Stemming from:*	Disease	43 (64)	58 (34)
		Family	14 (22)	37 (22)
		Hospital	43 (62)	5 (3)
Row 3	*Posed to:*	Nurse	27 (40)	21 (12)
		Family	47 (70)	64 (38)
		Doctor	9 (13)	
		Hospital	16 (24)	5 (3)
		Other	1 (1)	10 (6)
Row 4	*Emot/Tech:*	Tech	53 (79)	43 (26)
		Emot	20 (28)	34 (20)
		Admin	27 (41)	21 (12)
		Tech/Emot		2 (1)
Row 5	*Authority Reference:*	Nurse	63 (93)	32 (19)
		Doctor	24 (35)	35 (21)
		Family	5 (8)	12 (7)
		Hospital	7 (10)	21 (12)
		Other	1 (2)	
			N=148	N = 59

N = Number of problem units dealt with.

Table XXI

CROSSTABULATION OF DIABETIC CLINIC
(Value 1-1st Year)

Crtship	Smalltk Count Row Pct Col Pct	1	2	3	4	5	Row Total
	1	58	72	46	9	22	207
		28.0	34.8	22.2	4.3	10.6	10.6
		33.9	15.2	6.8	2.3	9.5	
	2	31	233	108	30	8	410
		7.6	56.8	26.3	7.3	2.0	21.0
		18.1	49.3	15.9	7.5	3.5	
	3	54	105	259	106	47	571
		9.5	18.4	45.4	18.6	8.2	29.3
		31.6	22.2	38.1	26.6	20.3	
	4	23	45	169	119	47	403
		5.7	11.2	41.9	29.5	11.7	20.6
		13.5	9.5	24.9	29.9	20.3	
	5	5	18	97	134	107	361
		1.4	5.0	26.9	37.1	29.6	18.5
		2.9	3.8	14.3	33.7	46.3	
	Column Total	171	473	679	398	231	1952
		8.8	24.2	34.8	20.4	11.8	100.0

Kendall's Tau B = 0.41073. Significance = 0.0
Kendall's Tau C = 0.39509. Significance = 0.0
ETA = 0.24084 with crtship dependent. = 0.22563 with Smalltk dependent.

Table XXII

CROSSTABULATION OF DIABETIC CLINIC
(Value 2-2nd Year)

Crtship	Count / Row Pct / Col Pct	Smalltk 1	2	3	4	5	Row Total
	1	103	394	171	61	3	732
		14.1	53.8	23.4	8.3	0.4	38.5
		66.5	51.5	28.0	17.7	12.5	
	2	41	286	175	68	2	572
		7.2	50.0	30.6	11.9	0.3	30.1
		26.5	37.4	28.6	19.7	8.3	
	3	8	72	192	129	7	408
		2.0	17.6	47.1	31.6	1.7	21.5
		5.2	9.4	31.4	37.4	29.2	
	4	3	13	71	79	10	176
		1.7	7.4	40.3	44.9	5.7	9.3
		1.9	1.7	11.6	22.9	41.7	
	5	0	0	2	8	2	12
		0.0	0.0	16.7	66.7	16.7	0.6
		0.0	0.0	0.3	2.3	8.3	
	Column Total	155	765	611	345	24	1900
		8.2	40.3	32.2	18.2	1.3	100.0

Kendall's Tau B = 0.39231. Significance = 0.0
Kendall's Tau C = 0.34348. Significance = 0.0
ETA=0.21996 with crtship dependent.=0.22278 with Smalltk dependent.
Number of missing observations=8

Table XXIII

CROSSTABULATION OF DIABETIC CLINIC
(Value 1-1st Year)

Crtship	Count Row Pct Col Pct	Oppfeed 1	2	3	4	5	Row Total
	1	166 80.2 11.9	2 1.0 18.2	6 2.9 3.0	8 3.9 5.4	25 12.1 12.9	207 10.6
	2	298 72.7 21.3	2 0.5 18.2	71 17.3 35.5	19 4.6 12.9	20 4.9 10.3	410 21.0
	3	391 68.5 27.9	3 0.5 27.3	61 10.7 30.5	55 9.6 37.4	61 10.7 31.4	571 29.3
	4	289 71.7 20.6	3 0.7 27.3	28 6.9 14.0	36 8.9 24.5	47 11.7 24.2	403 20.6
	5	256 70.9 18.3	1 0.3 9.1	34 9.4 17.0	29 8.0 19.7	41 11.4 21.1	361 18.5
	Column Total	1400 71.7	11 0.6	200 10.2	147 7.5	194 9.9	1952 100.0

Kendall's Tau B = 0.04213. Significance = 0.0026
Kendall's Tau C = 0.03157. Significance = 0.0183
ETA = 0.00561 with crtship dependent. = 0.00582 with oppfeed dependent.

Table XXIV

CROSSTABULATION OF DIABETIC CLINIC (Value 2-2nd Year)

Crtship	Count / Row Pct / Col Pct	Oppfeed 1	2	3	4	5	Row Total
	1	608	21	27	48	27	731
		83.2	2.9	3.7	6.6	3.7	38.5
		41.6	48.8	25.2	28.2	23.5	
	2	434	13	45	49	31	572
		75.9	2.3	7.9	8.6	5.4	30.1
		29.7	30.2	42.1	28.8	27.0	
	3	295	8	18	51	35	407
		72.5	2.0	4.4	12.5	8.6	21.4
		20.2	18.6	16.8	30.0	30.4	
	4	118	1	16	21	20	176
		67.0	0.6	9.1	11.9	11.4	9.3
		8.1	2.3	15.0	12.4	17.4	
	5	8	0	1	1	2	12
		66.7	0.0	8.3	8.3	16.7	0.6
		0.5	0.0	0.9	0.6	1.7	
	Column	1463	43	107	170	115	1893
	Total	77.1	2.3	5.6	9.0	6.1	100.0

Kendall's Tau B = 0.12188. Significance = 0.0000
Kendall's Tau C = 0.08000. Significance = 0.0000
ETA = 0.02454 with crtship dependent. = 0.02189 with Oppfeed dependent.
Number of missing observations = 10

Table XXV

CROSSTABULATION OF DIABETIC CLINIC (Value 1-1st Year)

Crtship	Service: Count / Row Pct / Col Pct	1	2	3	4	5	Row Total
	1	198	5	2	2	0	207
		95.7	2.4	1.0	1.0	0.0	10.6
		11.1	7.0	3.6	8.3	0.0	
	2	381	8	12	2	7	410
		92.9	2.0	2.9	0.5	1.7	21.0
		21.3	11.3	21.4	8.3	50.0	
	3	527	18	19	5	2	571
		92.3	3.2	3.3	0.9	0.4	29.3
		29.5	25.4	33.9	20.8	14.3	
	4	363	22	7	6	5	403
		90.1	5.5	1.7	1.5	1.2	20.6
		20.3	31.0	12.5	25.0	35.7	
	5	318	18	16	9	0	361
		88.1	5.0	4.4	2.5	0.0	18.5
		17.8	25.4	28.6	37.5	0.0	
	Column Total	1787	71	56	24	14	1952
		91.5	3.6	2.9	1.2	0.7	100.0

Kendall's Tau B = 0.06828. Significance = 0.0000
Kendall's Tau C = 0.03015. Significance = 0.0229
ETA = 0.00887 with crtship dependent. = 0.00453 with service dependent.

Table XXVI

CROSSTABULATION OF DIABETIC CLINIC (Value 2-2nd Year)

Crtship	Count / Row Pct / Col Pct	Service 1	2	3	4	5	Row Total
	1	689	30	7	6	0	732
		94.1	4.1	1.0	0.8	0.0	38.5
		41.0	27.0	11.5	16.2	0.0	
	2	489	53	18	10	2	572
		85.5	9.3	3.1	1.7	0.3	30.1
		29.1	47.7	29.5	27.0	20.0	
	3	344	15	29	14	6	408
		84.3	3.7	7.1	3.4	1.5	21.5
		20.5	13.5	47.5	37.8	60.0	
	4	149	11	7	7	2	176
		84.7	6.3	4.0	4.0	1.1	9.3
		8.9	9.9	11.5	18.9	20.0	
	5	10	2	0	0	0	12
		83.3	16.7	0.0	0.0	0.0	0.6
		0.6	1.8	0.0	0.0	0.0	
	Column Total	1681	111	61	37	10	1900
		88.5	5.8	3.2	1.9	0.5	100.0

Kendall's Tau B. = 0.12359. Significance = 0.0000
Kendall's Tau C = 0.05983. Significance = 0.0000
ETA = 0.02250 with crtship dependent. = 0.02609 with Service dependent.
Number of missing observations = 8

APPENDIX C

INSTRUMENTS

C-1. Check List Form

Beginning Time:
Ending Time:

ROLES PRESENT

(If more than one (1) are present in any category please indicate the number)

____ Clinic Nurse [CN]
____ Other Nurse [ON]
____ Patient [PT] ________ ____ ____
Age Sex
____ Physician [P] ________
____ Mother [M] ________
____ Father [F] ________

____ Clerk [C]
____ Technician [T]
____ Nursing Aid [NA]
____ Other [O] ________ (Specify)

Principal Opposite
Role Interacting
With Nurse ________

____ Other Adult Relative ________
____ Other Children ________ (number)

LOCATION

____ Waiting Room [WR] ____ Cast Room [CR] ____ Examination Room [ER]

____ Appointment and Record Desk [AD] ____ Other [O] ________ (Specify)

ACTIVITY

____ Health Teaching [HT] ____ Treatment [T] ____ Administrative [A]
OTHER [O] ________ (Specify)

C-2. Home Interview Questionnaire

Corresponding Clinic Tape Code Number: ______________________

Child's Full Name: ______________________
Address: ______________________

____
(Apt. No.)
____

Telephone No.: ______________________

If no Telephone, how to reach: ______________________

Interviewer: ______________________
Arranged for interview: through phone ______ Other ______________
Date of interview (day, month, hour): ______________________
Reason if interview could not be completed on appointed day:

Length of interview: ______ hour (s) ______ minutes
Condition of home:
_____ Good (Top 25% of neighborhood)
_____ Fair
_____ Poor (Lower 25% of neighborhood)

Race and Ethnicity:
_____ White
_____ Negro
_____ Puerto Rican
_____ Oriental
_____ Other

Does ______________________ like the nurses and doctors
(Name)
_____ Likes them very much
_____ Likes them some of the time
_____ Doesn't seem to care either way
_____ Is afraid of them
_____ Does not like them at all
_____ Likes the nurse(s), but not the doctor(s)
_____ Likes the doctor(s), but not the nurse(s)
_____ Other:

Does the nurse talk to you when you go there?
_____ Yes, very often
_____ Sometimes
_____ Very little
_____ Never
_____ Other:

Does the nurse talk more to you or to ______________________________?
(Name)

_____ More to Mother
_____ More to child
_____ Equally to both
_____ Nurse talks to neither
_____ Other:

Section II:

Now I would like to ask you some questions about the last time you went to the clinic:

When was your last visit to the clinic?

____

Whom did you see when you went there? (Do you remember their names?)

______________________ (Doctor)   ______________________ (Nurse)

What did you talk about with the doctor?

What did the doctor do for your child?

Do you think there was something the doctor should have done or should have told you, but didn't?

_____ Yes: (Explain) ______________________________
____

_____ No

Did the nurse give ______________ (Name) any tests the last time you were at the clinic

_____ Yes (If yes) What did she do?
_____ No

Did the nurse give you any advice about how to care for ______________ (Name)'s illness at home:

_____ Yes (Explain) What did she tell you to do?
_____ No

Has it been impossible to carry out any of the instructions the nurse gave you at the last visit to the clinic?

_____ Yes (Explain):
_____ No

Did you ask her any questions about what to do for the illness?

_____ Yes (Explain)
_____ No

Were you satisfied with the answers she gave you?

_____ Yes
_____ No (If No) Why not?

Did the nurse give ________________ (Name) any instructions about how to care for the illness?

_____ Yes (If Yes) What were these instructions?
_____ No

Did ________________ (Name) ask the nurse any questions about his illness or about what to do for it?

_____ Yes (If Yes) What did he ask and what did she answer?
_____ No

Were you and ________________ satisfied with her answers?

_____ Yes
_____ No (If No) Why not?

Do you think the visit really took care of all the problems and questions you had at that time?

_____ Yes
_____ No (If No) Why not?

Was there something you would have liked to have asked the doctor or the nurse the last time, but didn't?

_____ Yes (If Yes) Why didn't you ask then?
_____ No

How long did you have to wait the last time at the clinic?

____

Did you mind waiting or do you think you had to wait too long?

_____ Didn't mind waiting
_____ Waited too long
_____ Other:

How old is ________________ (Name)?

____

Section III:

(If child is six years or older, this section is to be included in the interview; if under six years, go to Section IV)

Now I'd like to ask you some questions about ________________ (Name):

How good is ________________ (Name) in following what the nurses and doctors tell him to do?

_____ Excellent
_____ Good
_____ Fair
_____ Poor

Does he do the things he is supposed to do about his illness?

_____ Always
_____ Often
_____ Sometimes
_____ Never

Is he able to follow the instructions when you're not around?
_____ Always
_____ Often
_____ Sometimes
_____ Never

Does he fail to do the things he should do for his illness?
_____ Always
_____ Often
_____ Sometimes
_____ Never

Section IV:

Now I'd like to ask some questions about the family in general:

Is ____ in school?
(Name)

How many children do you have all together? ____________________

How many people live here all together? ____________________

What is your husband's usual occupation?
______________________________ Employed presently? _____ Yes _____ No

How many years of schooling did your husband complete? ____________________

Could you estimate your total monthly income? ____________________

Do you rent or own your home?
_____ Rent
_____ Own

Residence:
_____ House
_____ Apartment

Number of rooms
_____ Large (6+ rooms)
_____ Medium (3-5 rooms)
_____ Small (1-2 rooms)

C-3. Code Book

VARIABLE LABELS		*Sub-category Labels*	
Col. 1	Clinics	1	Orthopedic
		2	Arthritis
		3	Diabetic
		4	Nutrition 1st year
		5	Scoleosis
		6	Nutrition 2nd year
		7	Med. Out-Pt.
Col. 2	Month	2	February
		3	March
		4	April
		6	June
		7	July
Col. 3	Date	0-3	
4		0-9	
Col. 5	Year	7	1st year
		8	2nd year
Col. 6	Family or Staff Number	001-013	Arthritis
7		100-208	Orthopedic
8		300-330	Diabetic
		400-438	Nutrition 1st year
		500-514	Scoleosis
		601-603	Nutrition 2nd year
		700-800	Med. Out-Pt.
		888	Fam. Unident.
		999	Staff only
Col. 9	Years of Age	0-2	
10		0-9	
11	Tenths of Year	0-9	
Col. 12	Sex of Child Interviewed	1	Male
		2	Female
Col. 13	No. of Children in Family	1-9	No. up to 9
		0	Staff only
Col. 14	Session	1	Morning
		2	Afternoon
Col. 15	Observer	1	7
		2	8
		3	9
		4	
		5	
		6	

Col. 16	Card Number	0-9	
17		0-9	
18		0-9	
19		0-9	
20		0-9	
Col. 21	Transcript Number	0-4	
22		0-9	
Col. 23	Transcript Page Number	0-4	
24		0-9	
Col. 25	Skip		
(PERSONS PRESENT COLUMNS)			
Col. 26	Nurse Present	0-1	
27	Doctor Present	0-1	
28	Mothers Present	0-9	
29	Patients Present	0-9	
30	Fathers Present	0-9	
31	Other Children Present	0-9	
32	Other Adult Fam. Present	0-9	
Col. 33	Other Nurses Present	0-9	
34	Other Doctors Present	0-9	
35	Clerk/Receptionist	0-9	
36	Aide	0-9	
Col. 37	Staff-Male-Unident.	0-9	
38	Staff-Female-Unident.	0-9	
39	Staff-Unidentified	0-9	
40	Other-Unknown	0-9	
Col. 41	Supervisor/Ph. Therapist	0-9	
42	Dietician	0-9	
43	Social Worker	0-9	
44	Clinic Chief	0-9	
Col. 45	Total Persons Present	0-9	(Count nos. of above)
46		0-9	
Col. 47	Communication	0	None
		1	Telephone
		2	Intercom
Col. 48	Location	1	Waiting Room
		2	Appoint Desk
		3	Corridor
		4	Exam Room
		5	Cast Room
		6	Nurse Office
		7	Outside Cl.
		8	Other
		9	Resident Rm.

Column	Variable	Code	Category	Note
Col. 49	Topic Ortho-Arthritis	01	Phys. Exam	
50		02	Treat/Exer.	
		03	Trt/Br-Ca-Cr	
		04	Treat/Drugs	
		05	Trt/Traction	
		06	Diet-Weight	
		07	Other Med.	
		08	Gen. Illness	
		09	Tape Rec.	
		10	Procedural	
		11	Referrals	
		12	Appointments	
		13	Hosp/Operat.	(Past, Present,
		14	Hosp/Operat.	Future)
		15	Holidays	
		16	Games/Activ.	
		17	School	
		18	Association	
		20	Socializing	
		23	Administrat.	
		24	Charts/Recs.	(Interstaff only)
		25	Rooms	
		26	Discuss Fam.	
Col. 51	Scope	1	Medical	
		2	Home	
		3	Life Cycle	
Col. 52	Skip			
53	Inquiring	0	None	
		2	What-mean?	
		2	Why-mean?	
		3	What-do?	
		4	Do-self?	
		5	Gen. Illness	
Col. 54	Predictive	0	None	
		1	If-Good/Bad	
		2	If-Explanat.	
		3	If-What do	
		4	If-Do self	
		5	Gen. Illness	
Col. 55	Other	0	None	(i.e. if either 53 or 54 (are punched 1-5)
		6	Other	(i.e. if 53 and 54 are 0)
Col. 56	Comments	0	None	
		1	Anxiety	
		2	Conflict	
		3	Support	
		4	Expect/Avoid	
		5	Explanation	
		6	Instruction	

		7 Tape 8 Other 9 Chief Resdnt
Col. 57 58	Bit/Lines per Initiation	0-9 0-9
Col. 59 60	Initiator	01-99
Col. 61 62	Recipient	01-99
Col. 63 64	Re	01-99
Col. 65	Greeting	1-4
Col. 66	Aggression	1-5
Col. 67	Small talk	1-5
Col. 68	Medical Information	1-5
Col. 69	Administration	1-5
Col. 70	Service	1-5
Col. 71	Opportunity for Feedback	1-5
Col. 72	Feedback	1-5
Col. 73	Self-Authority Reference	1-5
Col. 74	Other Authority Refer.	1-5
Col. 75	Pos./Neg. Authority Ref.	0 None (i.e. if 73 and 74 are 1) 1 Postitive (only if 73 and 74 2 Negative are punched 2-5)
Col. 76	Courtship	1-5
Col. 77	Humor	1-5
Col. 78	Parting	1-4
Col. 79	Inaudible/Incomplete	1 Inaud/Incomp 3 PrvSentinaud 4 FolSentinaud 5 Sent Muddled (before and after, i.e. should be two)

INDEX

P

R